MENINGEAL LEUKEMIA

MENINGEAL LEUKEMIA

Lawrence E. Broder, M. D.

and

Stephen K. Carter, M. D.

Cancer Therapy Evaluation Branch
National Cancer Institute
Bethesda, Maryland

ℚ SPRINGER SCIENCE+BUSINESS MEDIA, LLC · 1972

Library of Congress Catalog Card Number 74-190394

ISBN 978-1-4684-1991-7   ISBN 978-1-4684-1989-4 (eBook)
DOI 10.1007/978-1-4684-1989-4

© 1972 Springer Science+Business Media New York
Originally published by Plenum Pres, New York in 1972
Softcover reprint of the hardcover 1st edition 1972

CONTENTS

ACKNOWLEDGMENTS

We wish to thank Dr. C. Gordon Zubrod whose suggestion led to the inception of this book; Dr. David P. Rall who lent encouragement and useful suggestions in reviewing the book; and Mrs. Elsa Di Maria for her diligent work in the preparation of the manuscript. We also wish to acknowledge Mrs. Martha Harshman and Mrs. Rhonda Weinstein for typographical review of the manuscript.

I. INTRODUCTION

Meningeal leukemia (ML) is a well-known and rather frequent complication of leukemia especially since the advent of chemotherapy. The first report of neurological complications of leukemia was in 1823 by Burns[1]. Before leukemia chemotherapy, there had been only sporadic and relatively few case reports. However, since 1948, the incidence of meningeal leukemia has increased to where it is now one of the most frequent complications of the disease.

This review will discuss in depth the pathology, clinical characteristics, and results of treatment of meningeal leukemia. An attempt will be made to assess the relative values of different modes of therapy and suggest new ones in light of animal studies and theoretical models for meningeal leukemia, and to define what parameters are necessary in evaluating the results of therapy, which would be helpful in future studies. This is especially cogent since many of the more recent chemotherapy protocols are utilizing combinations of radiotherapy and intrathecal therapy both in treatment of meningeal leukemia and as prophylaxis against its development.

The format of this review involves an individual discussion of the drugs or methods of therapy of meningeal leukemia. Tables have been made which summarize the individual reports. On those tables are listed key factors which appear to play a role in the treatment of meningeal leukemia. Such factors include the age, hematological status, number of episodes, treatment, response (both subjective and objective when available), duration of central nervous system (CNS) remission, and some survival data when available.

From these more extensive tables, summaries of the above factors have been derived. These have been discussed separately in the section entitled Characteristics of Meningeal Leukemia. In that section data has been collected from the individual reports on pathology, incidence, occurrence, development, episodes, male-female incidence, and hematological status of patients with meningeal leukemia. An entire chapter has also been devoted to assessing the various signs and symptoms in terms of frequency and prognosis.

Therapy using parenteral or oral drug administration is discussed next. This chapter is followed by a discussion of BCNU therapy and pyrimethamine therapy for meningeal leukemia since these agents are known to cross the blood brain barrier and affect the course of meningeal disease.

Intrathecal therapy is discussed as a whole with sub-sections reserved for discussions of individual drugs.

The treatment of meningeal leukemia by radiotherapy is then outlined, followed by a discussion of the combination of chemotherapy and radiotherapy. The last chapters involve an overview of the treatment of leukemia in general and the role of CNS prophylaxis therapy in this treatment.

REFERENCES

1. Burns, A. Observations on the surgical anatomy of the head and neck. Baltimore, F. Lucas, Jr., E.J. Coale, and Cushing & Jewett, 1823.

II. CHARACTERISTICS OF MENINGEAL LEUKEMIA

A. Pathology

Meningeal leukemia is a clinical syndrome encompassing a number of symptoms and signs which are related to CNS involvement by either leukemic infiltration or the secondary effects of the systemic disease. Leukemic infiltration and intracranial hemorrhage appear to be the most common mechanisms by which the syndrome is produced. In this section the early literature on the pathological involvement of the CNS by leukemia will be reviewed and compared with some recent clinico-pathological reports.

There have been many reports of leukemic involvement of the central nervous system since Burns[1] in 1823 described a strange growth in the brain due to a case of cerebral chloroma. In a literature review of 38 cases of chloroma by Dock and Warthin in 1904[2], 14 cases of cerebral and spinal involvement were described. In 1926, Fried[3] summarized 30 cases and added one case of his own. Lesions of the nervous system were found in the hemispheres in twelve, in the cranial nerves in eight, and in the cord in eleven cases. In 1927, Tromner and Wohlwill[4] reported 12 cases of leukemia with neurological complications in 9 of these. At necropsy, 11 of the 12 cases (91%) had microscopic evidence of invasion of the central nervous system. In 1934, Diamond[5] described 14 cases of leukemia with cerebral involvement. The leukemia types included 5 myelogenous, 4 lymphatic, 2 myeloblastic, 2 stem cell, and one monocytic in type. In all cases he described infiltration of the pia mater and perivascular spaces. In addition, the author believed that infiltration around the chiasma could give rise to papilledema.

TABLE I
Neurologic Lesions in 146 Cases of Leukemia Reported in the
Literature[6]

Type of lesion	No. of cases	Per cent of total
Cranial meninges	26	17.8
Cranial nerve nuclei	23	15.7
Cerebral invasion	23	15.7
Cerebral hemorrhage	47	32.2
Peripheral nerve	2	1.4
Spinal meninges	10	6.9
Spinal cord invasion	12	8.2
Spinal cord hemorrhage	1	0.7
Spinal extradural	2	1.4
Total	146	100.0

TABLE II
Neurological Symptoms and Signs in 69 Cases of Leukemia Recorded in
three Boston Hospitals[6]

Clinical manifestations	No. of cases	Per cent of total
Cranial nerve palsies or anesthesia	21	30
Absent reflexes	13	19
Pyramidal signs	8	12
Paresthesias	10	14
Herpes	4	6
Meningeal signs	5	7
Miscellaneous: Coma, paralysis, tremors	8	12
Total	69	100

In 1935, Schwab and Weiss[6] reviewed the above reports
as well as other case reports described in the literature
from 1835 to 1935. These totaled 146 cases reported by
75 authors. The type of neurologic lesion reported in those
cases which came to postmortem examination are shown in
Table I. Of the 23 cases with cranial nerve involvement,
17 involved the seventh nerve, and 7 involved the sixth
nerve. The eight, ninth, tenth, eleventh, and twelfth
cranial nerves were the least frequently involved.

In addition to the case reports reviewed, Schwab and
Weiss[6] analyzed, for neurologic signs and symptoms, 334
cases of leukemia recorded in three Boston Hospitals. It
was found that 20.5% had neurologic complications. The
types of neurological complications in these 69 cases are
described in Table II. It is of interest that the most
frequent neurologic manifestations were cranial nerve
palsies or anesthesias. As will be seen in the section
on signs and symptoms in this review, the frequency of
occurrence of cranial nerve signs (30%) is not far from
the 22% frequency found in the present review.

TABLE III
Neurologic Involvement in Different Types of Leukemia[6]

Type of leukemia	Total cases		Involvement of central nervous system		Retinal Involvement	
	No.	%	No.	%	No.	%
Three Boston hospitals (334 cases)						
Acute lymphatic	62	18.5	14	22.6	14	22.6
Chronic lymphatic	80	23.9	17	21.2	8	10.0
Acute myelogenous	58	17.3	13	22.4	8	13.8
Chronic myelogenous	91	27.2	21	23.1	7	7.7
Miscellaneous group	43	12.9	4	9.3	1	2.3

In the 334 cases analyzed by Schwab and Weiss[6] there was an equal occurrence of neurologic manifestations in all types of leukemia (see Table III). This result is interesting since in our review, the majority of patients with CNS manifestations were patients with acute lymphocytic leukemia (ALL).

In the Schwab and Weiss[6] review, analysis of the results of spinal fluid determinations were accomplished in ten of 146 patients with CNS leukemia described in the literature and in an additional 10 of 334 patients whose case records were reviewed from three Boston hospitals. Of this total of 34 cases available, only nine (26.4%) had normal spinal fluids. The most frequent abnormalities on the cerebrospinal fluid were in the protein content (in 52.9%), the pressure (in 35.3%) and the cell content (in 41.4%). In our series reported under the section on signs and symptoms, just the opposite results were seen. The presence of cells and an elevated CSF pressure were found in ≈ 90% of the cases whereas an elevated CSF protein was found in less than 50% of the cases.

The Schwab and Weiss[6] report was limited in that only 3.3% of the 334 patients had postmortem examinations of the central nervous system. Thus, overall pathological involvement of the CNS in the total patients with leukemia is lacking. A more recent study by Leidler and Russell[7], in 1945, revealed that in 20 patients with leukemia examined for meningeal involvement, such involvement was found in ≈ 90% of patients. Their principal findings included (1) hemorrhage and leukemic infiltration in the meninges, (2) hemorrhage and leukemic infiltration in the brain, (3) leukemic infiltration, per se, in the brain, and (4) leukostasis. Pathological changes were also noted in the neuronal, supportive, and vascular elements of the brain but these were usually associated with infiltration, hemorrhage, or both. They concluded that 80% of leukemic patients have significant pathological changes in the brain but that only 20-35% of these patients have neurologic symptoms or signs. It thus becomes evident that in the years before the onset of chemotherapy, many patients with CNS involvement by leukemia exhibited leukemic infiltrations and/or intracranial hemorrhages as the primary pathological characteristics.

That this same pathological pattern has persisted after the advent of chemotherapy has been elucidated by a number of clinico-pathological reports. Hunt, in 1959[8] described the neurologic complications in 815 patients with various types of leukemia. In this group there were 18% Acute Lymphocytic Leukemia (ALL), 37% Chronic Lymphocytic Leukemia (CLL), 6% Acute Myelocytic Leukemia (AML), 21% Chronic Myelocytic Leukemia (CML), 18% Acute Myelo- Monocytic Leukemia (AMoL). Of those patients that were followed, there were 86 patients who died of hemorrhage into the

CNS and 15 patients had leukemic infiltrations. The usual pattern was massive intracerebral, subarachnoid, or intra-axial hemorrhage, associated with severe thrombocytopenia, usually with clinical evidence of hemorrhagic diathesis elsewhere. There were few instances of subdural hematoma. They described several "clinical types" of pathological involvement by leukemic cells. The most important variant they considered to be the "Hydrops pattern" which was present in 11/15 patients and included the presence of severe increase in intracranial pressure due to swollen brain. Hydrocephalus, secondary to leukemic infiltration, accounted for one of the complications in their 15 cases. The third characteristic which they described was intra-axial and perineural infiltration in the peripheral nerves, which occurred in one patient.

Moore and his colleagues[9] reviewed the pathological findings in 117 cases of acute leukemia treated at the National Cancer Institute. Intracranial hemorrhage was responsible for death in 20%. The majority of fatal intra-cerebral hemorrhages occurred most frequently in those patients in which the frequency of intracerebral leuco-stasis and leukemic nodules were high. In contrast, fatal subarachnoid hemorrhages were not associated with these findings and appeared to be related to severe thrombocy-topenia. Leukemic infiltration of the dura was noted in 70% of patients with lymphocytic leukemia and in 59% of patients with myelocytic leukemia. In contrast to the high incidence of dural involvement, leukemic infiltration of the arachnoid was found in only 30% of the 117 cases. Perivascular infiltration or cuffing was observed in only 19% of the cases. Seventy five per cent of patients with either arachnoid or perivascular infiltration of the meninges demonstrated hydrocephalus.

As we shall see in the next section, whereas the incidence of meningeal leukemia has increased, the patho-logicial features of the syndrome appear to have been un-changed by the advent of chemotherapy.

REFERENCES

1. Burns, A. Observations on the surgical anatomy of the head and neck. Baltimore, F. Lucas, Jr., E.J. Coale, and Cushing & Jewett, 1823.

2. Dock, G., and Warthin, A.S. New case of chloroma with leukemia; with a study of cases reported since 1893. Trans Ass Amer Physicians, 19: 64, 1904.

3. Fried, B.M. Leukemia and the central nervous system with review of 30 cases. Arch Path Lab Med 2: 23, 1926.

4. Tromner, E., and Wohlwill, F. Uber erkrankungen des nervensystems, insbesondere der hirnnerven, bei leukamie. Disch Z. Nervenheilk 100: 233, 1927.

5. Diamond, I.B. Leukemic changes in the brain. A report of fourteen cases. Arch Neurol Psychiat 32: 118, 1934.

6. Schwab, R.S., and Weiss, S. The neurologic aspect of leukemia. Amer J Med Sci 189: 766, 1935.

7. Leidler, F., and Russell, W.O. The brain in leukemia. A clinico-pathologic study of twenty cases with a review of the literature. Arch Path 40: 14, 1945.

8. Hunt, W.E., Bouroncle, B.A., and Meagher, J.N. Neurologic complications of leukemias and lymphomas. J Neurosurg 16: 135, 1959.

9. Moore, E.W., Thomas, L.B., Shaw, R.K., and Freireich, E.J. The central nervous system in acute leukemia, AMA. Arch Intern Med 105: 141, 1960.

B. Incidence, Occurrence, Development

1. Incidence

This review describes the published data on patients with ML that have been treated with either chemotherapy or radiotherapy since about 1948. A historical review of a few of the reports of meningeal leukemia before about 1948 have been included for incidence comparisons.

As can be seen from Table I, the incidence of meningeal leukemia before the advent of chemotherapy varied anywhere from 2% to ≃ 75.0%. One reason for this variation may be attributed to the inclusion, in many of the series, of CNS complications due to the systemic disease. There were patients for example with hemorrhage due to thrombocytopenia. The comparison between the incidence in these earlier series and the more recent series is therefore difficult to evaluate.

In contrast to the period before chemotherapy, more recent series have delineated between the complications of meningeal leukemia, per se, and that due to the systemic disease. It is from these series that we can obtain a relatively accurate assessment of the trend in the incidence of meningeal leukemia. As can be seen in Table II, there appears to be a significant difference between the incidence of meningeal leukemia in the decade before 1960 and that after it.

Indeed in the space of ≃ 10 years the incidence has risen about 2 1/2 times. Several series such as Evans[9] have even compared the incidence according to year. Evans found about a ten-fold increase in the incidence of

TABLE I
Incidence of Meningeal Leukemia
Prior to Chemotherapy

Year	Reference	Incidence (%)	Remarks
1921	Bass[1]	26	All types of CNS involvement
1927	Tromner and Wohlwill[2]	75	11/12 at necropsy (92%)
1934	Diamond[3]	28.5	
1935	Schwab and Weiss[4]	20.5	Only meningeal involvement
1943	Kirshbaum and Preuss[5]	10	
1945	Leidler and Russell[6]	20-35	Neurological signs and symptoms
1945	Brandt[7]	9	
1947	Sparling et al[8]	20	

TABLE II
Incidence of Meningeal Leukemia
After Advent of Chemotherapy

Year	Reference	Total # Patients	Total # ML Patients	Incidence (%)
1947-60	Evans (1963)[9]	915	151	16.8
1953-58	Shaw et al (1960)[10]	150	25	16.7
1954-57	Hunt et al (1959)[11]	815	15	1.8
1952-60	Pierce (1962)[12]	232	26	11.0
1953-57	D'Angio et al (1959)[13]	372	37	9.9
Incidence to 1960		2484	254	10.2
1954-64	Koch et al (1966)[14]	192	28	14.6
1955-64	Haghbin and Zuelzer (1965)[15]	285	61	21.4
1958-66	Hardisty and Norman (1967)[16]	131	29	22.0
1961-63	Nies et al (1965)[17]	99	27	27.0
1963-64	Evans et al (1970)[18]	209	106	51.0
1965	Frei et al (1965)[19]	106	10	9.4
1968	George et al (1968)[20]	31	13	42.0
1968	Falkson et al (1969)[21]	39	12	30.0
Incidence 1960 on		1165	299	25.6
Overall Incidence		3649	553	15.2

meningeal leukemia (from 4% to 40%) between 1947 and 1960. In a more recent series by the same author the incidence of meningeal leukemia from 1963-1964 was 51%[18]. It seems valid to apply the Chi-square statistical evaluation to this latter study since one can be reasonably assured that the patients were similarly evaluated. Thus the data of Table III are obtained with the differences between the two studies being highly significant.

TABLE III

Evans[9,18]	Incidence to 1960 (1947-1960)	Incidence from 1960 (1964-)	Total
+	151	106	257
-	764	103	867
Total	915	209	1124

$X^2 = 111.0$ or $p < .000001$

Apparently, increased awareness of the syndrome is no doubt contributing to the higher incidence figures being reported at least in some series. Diagnosis of the complication was more frequent in the Nies'[17] second series, for example, because routine lumbar punctures were done and abnormalities detected in asymptomatic patients.

Increased survival of patients may also play a role in the increased incidence of meningeal leukemia. In Evan's earlier series[9], the incidence of meningeal leukemia increased from 3-40% as the median survival rose 4-12 months. In her later series[18], encompassing patients treated between 1963-1964 and where the incidence of CNS leukemia was 51%, the median survival was 18 months.

That increased survival may be the key factor is supported by animal experiments. It has been shown that as one delays methotrexate (MTX) treatment of a mouse with intraperitoneally (IP) inoculated L1210 leukemia, the survival of the mouse is increased[22]. Concomitant with the lengthening of survival, the incidence of meningeal and cerebral infiltration by leukemic cells increases proportionally.

Another possibility for the increased incidence may be utilization of newer drugs and combinations of drugs. Indeed at the National Cancer Institute, the survival of patients with leukemia increased dramatically when combinations of drugs were utilized. Also, one major difference between the decades 1950-1960 and 1960-1970 was the increased use of new drug combinations in the treatment of leukemia.

2. Episodes

As the survival time increases in man, one may expect more time for the development of meningeal leukemia. Indeed, it is usually the case that patients who survive the first episode of CNS leukemia may have recurrence of the disease at a later date. In this review we have evaluated several large series to determine data in regards to the number of episodes of meningeal leukemia per patient. This data is shown in Table IV. Only those series where the number of episodes was specifically recorded were evaluated.

There were 1134 episodes of the clinical syndrome in the 535 cases that could be evaluated for number of episodes. This represents ≈ 2.0 episodes for each patient. The median time to the development of the first episode was ≈ 9.5 months. Others have confirmed this time to the first occurrence of the disease. In Hardisty and Norman's report[16], 28 episodes occurred after the median time to the first episode, while 22 occurred before. This suggests an in-

TABLE IV
Episodes of Meningeal Leukemia per Patient

Reference	Total # Pts. with Leukemia	Total # Pts. with ML	Total # Episodes of ML	Duration of Leukemia before CNS Disease (Mos.)
Evans[9]	921	151	315	
Shaw et al[10]	150	25	31	7.0
Hyman et al[23]	59	59	109	
Koch et al[14]	192	28	44	22.0
Hardisty & Norman[16]	131	29	50	9.5
Haghbin & Zuelzer[15]	285	61	164	12.3
Nies et al[17]	99	27	38	
Falkson et al[21]	39	12	17	7.0
D'Angio et al[13]	372	37	86	9.0
Evans et al[18]	209	106	280	9.0
Total	2457	535	1134	median 9.5

creasing number of episodes in those patients who survived longer than $\approx$ 10 months.

3. Pattern of Occurrence

Many have attempted to evaluate a pattern to the occurrence of CNS leukemia. This could be variable due to differing philosphies of the individual investigators concerning routine spinal taps. It has been shown, for example, that meningeal leukemia could be present without symptoms both in postmortem studies and in antemortem cytological examination of the spinal fluid. Hyman et al[23] found in their study of 34 patients with meningeal leukemia that CNS involvement developed uncommonly during the first three months of the disease; but after this period, there was a sharp increase in incidence so that half the cases were recognized by seven months after the diagnosis. In the Shaw et al study[10], only eight of the 21 patients with meningeal leukemia had the syndrome within four months of the onset of leukemia. Evans[9] found in 151 patients with meningeal leukemia that CNS involvement occurred at any stage of the disease from the time of diagnosis to the eighty-sixth month thereafter. The rate of involvement varied from 1.2% during the first three months after the diagnosis to 2.5% between 21 and 23 months from the diagnosis. In addition, their data showed that those children who developed CNS symptoms sometime in the course of the disease actually lived longer than those who did not. Since those patients who have a longer survival may have a greater tendency to develop CNS symptoms at some time in their course, this is understandable.

Hardisty and Norman[16] analyzed this point further. They found that meningeal leukemia occurred with fairly constant frequency throughout the first 18 months after the original diagnosis; although in two instances, meningeal involvement occurred within the first 8 weeks. About 4 of their 29 cases developed meningeal leukemia within the first three months. They further pointed out that, as would be expected of a complication which is likely to occur at any stage of the disease, the incidence of meningeal leukemia increases as the patient's overall survival is prolonged. They felt that meningeal involvement is usually a late complication, in the sense that it tends to develop towards the end of a patient's course. Those who developed meningeal leukemia early, with few exceptions, were among the short survivors.

4. Male - Female Incidence

Leidler and Russell[6] found neurological complications to occur twice as frequently in males than in females. Wells[24] found no significant difference in the incidence between the two sexes. The approximate incidence between the sexes probably lies somewhere between these two extremes. There were only three studies where the male-female ratio of systemic leukemia could be directly compared with the sex ratio in those patients developing CNS leukemia. This is given in Table V. The ratio of males to females who developed CNS leukemia is about equal to the ratio of males to females in the population of patients with systemic disease.

5. Patterns of Development

It becomes immediately apparent when reviewing the frequency of patients with various types of systemic leukemia, that the development of CNS manifestations is not proportional to the reported frequencies of systemic leukemia. Wintrobe[25] found that in $\simeq$ 3,000 cases of leukemia that he reviewed, $\simeq$ 28% were CLL, 26.6% were

TABLE V
Incidence of Meningeal Leukemia by Sex

Reference	Systemic Leukemia		CNS Leukemia	
	Male	Female	Male	Female
Shaw et al[10]	96	54	22	3
Koch et al[14]	97	95	18	23
Evans et al[18]	111	98	60	46
Total	304	247	100	72
Percent of total	55%	45%	58%	42%

CML, 20.0% were ALL, 16.9% were AML, and ≈ 7.8% were AMoL.
It is also interesting to note that ≈ 90% of all cases of
CLL or CML are adults and that ≈ 50% of the cases of AML
are adults. Thus, if the incidence of meningeal leukemia
paralleled the incidence of various systemic leukemias,
one would expect at least 50% of those patients with meningeal leukemia to be either adults or have CLL or CML.
That these parallels do not hold up when one evaluates the
characteristics of those patients with CNS leukemia is apparent from the following data. In this review of the patients with meningeal leukemia whose leukemia type was
reported, more than 90% had ALL while about 10% had AML
or blast crisis of CML. Thus, the great majority
of patients with CNS leukemia have ALL. The incidence is
about 4 times more than the incidence of ALL in the leukemia
population. Also in this review, only 18 adults have been
described with the syndrome (≈ 2.3%). This is very much
less than the incidence of adults with leukemia in the
leukemia population. Of the 18 adults in this series that
were reported to have meningeal leukemia, 9 had ALL and 7
had AML. It is interesting that there were two additional
patients in whom CNS leukemia developed as a manifestation
of metamorphosis from CML to AML. Adults generally do not
respond well to systemic therapy and therefore die early.
For this reason, perhaps, the incidence of meningeal leukemia is less.

6. Hematological Status

In this review of the patients with meningeal leukemia
(ALL), there were 235 patients in which the hematological
status of the patient was stated. Of these, 116 of the
patients were in complete remission and 113 were in relapse
at the time of the CNS manifestations. In three series, 6
partial remissions were listed. Of the adults (18 patients)
9 were in complete remission and 4 were in relapse. The
status of 5 patients was not given. Of the adults, two of
the four in relapse were in blastic metamorphosis of CGL.

Almost invariably most of the patients were on some
form of anti-leukemia systemic therapy either to induce
remissions or as maintenance with various combinations of
steroids (prednisone), antimetabolites (6-MP, methotrexate,
aminopterin) vinca alkaloids (vincristine, vinblastine),
S-phase inhibitors (cytosine arabinoside), antibiotics
(daunomycin), and alkylating agents (cyclophosphamide).
There is very little data concerning the effect of a particular antimetabolite or other cancer chemotherapy on
the occurrence of meningeal leukemia.

A few of the reports mentioned the concomitant use of
cancer chemotherapy agents, but when mentioned it is often
done in passing. Hardisty and Norman[24], however, evaluated
this point specifically in 50 episodes of meningeal leukemia in 29 patients. All patients were being treated with

an antimetabolite at the time of diagnosis of meningeal
involvement and nine were also receiving adrenocortical
steroids. There was no particular tendency for CNS leukemia to develop during the administration of any one
chemotherapeutic agent: 18 episodes occurred in patients
receiving 6-MP, 17 during methotrexate therapy, eight
while the patient was on cyclophosphamide, and seven
while on vincristine.

The sum total of the patients in hematological remission, at one point in time, should have a longer median survival than a similar group of patients who were in hematological relapse, for a certain percentage of patients
will resist induction into remission. In Hardisty and
Norman's series[16] in the leukemic population from which
the patients with meningeal leukemia were drawn, it was
observed that the median duration of the first remission,
and the median over-all survival, were significantly longer
for patients with less than 10,000 blasts/per mm^3 peripheral blood at diagnosis than those with more than this.
A comparison of CSF and blood counts in these patients
was therefore carried out and revealed a significant association between CSF cell count at diagnosis of each episode
of meningeal leukemia and the number of blasts in the
peripheral blood at the time of initial diagnosis of
leukemia. Melhor[26] also demonstrated the association between the peripheral white blood count and the occurrence
of CNS involvement. He did a randomized controlled study
of the use of prophylactic IT methotrexate in the preven-
tion of meningeal leukemia. Furthermore, he divided his
patients according to their peripheral white blood cell
counts at the time of original diagnosis. Among 23 patients
with initial WBC less than 10,000/mm^3, 10 (43.5%) developed CNS infiltration. In 20 patients with WBC greater than
10,000/mm^3, 16 (80.0%) showed CNS involvement. This difference was highly significant.

In animal studies utilizing bioassay techniques done
by Skipper and Schabel[27], it has been shown that the entry
of leukemic cells into the brain of a mouse occurs only
when the host's leukemic population is on the order of
10^7 cells. Apparently then, relapse, such as is occurring
at the first manifestation of the disease, may ultimately
affect the severity of meningeal involvement at a later
time. Pierce et al[12], found that when the meningeal complication develops during a hematologic relapse, transient
improvement in the meningeal signs and symptoms may be
obtained with either irradiation or intrathecal antifolic
drugs, but recurrence of the meningeal signs is common,
and life expectancy shortened.

As will be discussed in the next several sections,
the inability of some of these drugs used systemically to
cross the "blood-brain barrier" may play a role in the
development of meningeal leukemia. Shaw[10] found that of

twenty five patients with CNS leukemia, 17 had no further
hematologic remissions while the remaining eight patients
had either a complete or partial remission. Concomitant
neurologic improvement uncomplicated by whole brain irradiation or intrathecal (IT) methotrexate occurred in six
of these patients while on systemic antileukemic therapy.
However, of the 17 patients who failed to achieve another
hematological remission, only two demonstrated neurological
improvement, which in both was of short duration. Thus,
neurologic improvement with systemic chemotherapy occurs
primarily when a systemic remission occurs (P = <0.01).

In summary then, it can be stated that meningeal leukemia occurs primarily in children with acute lymphoblastic
leukemia. It is more common in males than females basically
because there is a higher incidence of males in the leukemia population. It can occur at any time. However, of
those who will develop CNS manifestations of leukemia
(30% of cases), about half of them will develop the meningeal leukemia by nine months after the onset of the disease. Generally as the survival in acute leukemia is
lengthened by chemotherapeutic agents the incidence of
meningeal complications tends to rise.

Almost invariably, since the advent of chemotherapy,
those patients who developed ML were on some form of antileukemic systemic therapy at the time. In our review,
≈ 55% of patients were in systemic remission while 45%
were in relapse when the meningeal leukemia developed.
Hematological relapse at the time of development of meningeal leukemia portends a poorer prognosis.

REFERENCES

1. Bass, M.H. Leukemia in children with special reference to lesions in the nervous system. Amer J Med
   Sci 162: 647, 1921.

2. Tromner, E., and Wohlwill, F. Uber erkrankugen des
   nervensystems, insbesondere der hirnnerven, bei
   leukamie. Disch Z. Nervenheilk 100: 233, 1927.

3. Diamond, I.B. Leukemic changes in the brain. A report
   of fourteen cases. Arch Neurol Psychiat 32: 118, 1934.

4. Schwab, R.S., and Weiss, S. The neurologic aspect of
   leukemia. Amer J Med Sci 189: 766, 1935.

5. Kirshbaum, J.D., and Preuss, F.S. Leukemia. A clinical
   and pathologic study of one hundred and twenty-three
   fatal cases in a series of 14,400 necropsies, AMA.
   Arch Intern Med 71: 777, 1953.

6. Leidler, F., and Russell, W.O. The brain in leukemia.
   A clinico-pathologic study of twenty cases with a
   review of the literature. Arch Path 40: 14, 1945.

7. Brandt, S. Alterations leucemiques de systeme nerveux.
   Acta Psychiat Neurol 20: 107, 1945.

8. Sparling, H.J. Adams, R.D., and Parker, F., Jr.
   Involvement of the nervous system by malignant lymphoma.
   Medicine 26: 285, 1947.

9. Evans, A.E. Central nervous system involvement in
   children with acute leukemia. Cancer 17: 256, 1963.

10. Shaw, R.K., Moore, E.W., Freireich, E.J., and Thomas,
    L.B. Meningeal leukemia. A syndrome resulting from
    increased intracranial pressure in patients with acute
    leukemia. Neurology 10: 823, 1960.

11. Hunt, W.E., Bouroncle, B.A., and Meagher, J.N. Neuro-
    logic complications of leukemias and lymphomas. J
    Neurosurg 16: 135, 1959.

12. Pierce, M.I. Neurologic complications in acute leuke-
    mia in children. Pediat Clin N Amer 9: 425, 1962.

13. D'Angio, G.J., Evans, A.E., and Mitus, A. Roentgen
    therapy of certain complications of acute leukemia
    in childhood. Amer J Roentgen 82: 541, 1959.

14. Koch, K., Reiquam, C.W., and Beatty, E.C., Jr. Acute
    childhood leukemia. Unusual complications. Rocky
    Mountain Med J 63: 50, 1966.

15. Haghbin, M., and Zuelzer, W.W. A long-term study of
    cerebrospinal leukemia. J Pediat 67: 23, 1965.

16. Hardisty, R.M., and Norman, P.M. Meningeal leukaemia
    Arch Dis Child 42:411, 1967.

17. Nies, B.A., Thomas, L.B., and Freireich, E.J. Menin-
    geal leukemia, a follow-up study. Cancer 18(5): 546,
    1965.

18. Evans, A.E., Gilbert, E.S., and Zandstra, R. The in-
    creasing incidence of central nervous system leukemia
    in children (Children's Cancer Study Group A). Cancer
    26: 404, 1970.

19. Frei, E. III, et al. The effectiveness of combinations
    of antileukemic agents in inducing and maintaining
    remission in children with acute leukemia. Blood
    26(5): 642, 1965.

20. George, P., Hernandez, K., Hustu, O., Borella, L., Holton, C., Pinkel, D. A study of "total therapy" of acute lymphocytic leukemia in children. Pediat Pharmacol Ther 72: 399, 1968.

21. Falkson, G., Van Eden, E.B., and Falkson, H.C. Meningeal leukaemia. Med Proc Johannesburg 15: 13, 1968.

22. Thomas, L.B., Chirigos, M.A., Humphreys, S.R., and Goldin, A. Development of meningeal leukemia (L1210) during treatment of subcutaneously inoculated mice with methotrexate. Cancer 17(3): 352, 1964.

23. Hyman, C.B., Bogle, J.M. Brubaker, C.A., Williams, K., and Hammond, D. Central nervous system involvement by leukemia in children. II. Therapy with intrathecal methotrexate. Blood 25: 13, 1965.

24. Wells, C.E., and Silver, R.T. The neurologic manifestations of the acute leukemias. A clinical study. Ann Intern Med 46: 439, 1957.

25. Wintrobe, M.M. Clinical hematology. Philadelphia, Lea and Febiger, 1967.

26. Melhorn, D.K., Gross, S., Fisher, B.J., and Newman, A.J. Studies on the use of "prophylactic" intrathecal amethopterin in childhood leukemia. Blood 36: 55, 1970.

27. Skipper, H.E., Schabel, F.M., Jr., and Wilcox, W.S. XIII. On the criteria and kinetics associated with "curability" of experimental leukemia. Cancer Chemother Rep 35: 1, 964.

C. Signs and Symptoms

From a review of the incidences of the various symptoms of CNS leukemia, nausea and vomiting and headache are by far the most common symptoms. As can be seen in Table I, nausea and vomiting were seen in ≃ 63% of the patients in which the symptoms of the cases were listed. Headache occurred in ≃ 61% of the cases. These symptoms have been ascribed to increasing CSF pressure. Other symptoms that occurred, although less common, included lethargy in ≃ 35% of the cases in which this symptom was listed. Ocular manifestations, such as diplopia, blindness, strabismus and blurred vision, occurred variably ranging from an incidence of ≃ 3% to ≃ 44% with an average of ≃ 20%. Hyman et al[8], in the review of his experience with meningeal leukemia, mentioned a 20% incidence of psychological disturbances which included hyperirritability, hallucinations, catatonic depression and disorientation. Vertigo occurred in ≃ 15% of his cases. Convulsions which could be a manifestation of increased intracranial pressure, as well as leukemic infiltration of the cerebrum, or meningeal irritation, was present in ≃ 15% of the cases. Coma was mentioned as occurring in ≃ 4 to 44% of the patients with an average of ≃ 17%. Other symptoms which were mentioned were irritability in ≃ 20%, abdominal pain in ≃ 7%, Cheyne-Stokes respiration in ≃ 7% and an auditory disturbance in ≃ 9%.

Generally the signs seen in meningeal leukemia (See Table II), like the symptoms, can be categorized as to pathogenesis. Among those signs which are due to increassing intracranial pressure, papilledema was the most frequent occurring in ≃ 49% of the cases. Suture separation occurred in ≃ 34% of the patients and was not present in the adults. Frank hydrocephalus, however, was only mentioned in one series and there the incidence was only 7%.

Facial palsy, which could be both a manifestation of increasing intracranial pressure or due to leukemia infiltration of the nerve roots, was mentioned in all the series polled and occurred with an incidence of ≃ 22%. Generally, when the cranial nerves are involved, the seventh is most common, then the second, eighth, and third in that order of frequency[10]. Peripheral nerve palsy occurred less commonly, being mentioned in only four of the reports polled and occurred in ≃ 5% of the cases.

Some have stated that involvement of the spinal cord and roots seems to be more common in the myelogenous form of leukemia than in the lymphatic form of the disease[10]. Sullivan[11] reported three interesting cases out of a series of 32. These three patients presented with spinal nerve involvement by leukemia in the form of weakness and/or pain in the lower extremities. Postmortem studies revealed a mild to intense leukemic infiltration of the cerebral and spinal meninges, spinal nerves, nerve roots, and perivascular spaces. The patients responded to IT methotrexate. All 3 had the ALL form of the disease.

CNS leukemia mimicking multifocal leukoencephalopathy has been reported[12]. The patient was a four year old boy who had tremor, ataxia, and transient hemiparesis without classic signs of meningeal irritation. Lumbar puncture revealed normal pressure but elevated WBC ($7760/mm^3$), elevated protein (200 mg/100 ml) and decreased sugar concentration (22 mg/100 ml). The patient responded to IT methotrexate.

Other signs which may be attributed to CNS infiltration by leukemic cells were found less occasionally. Reflex changes were reported in only one series and the incidence here was 40%. Pupillary changes were reported in $\simeq$ 20% of the cases while the Babinski's sign was reported in $\simeq$ 32% of cases in Shaw's report[1]. Auditory and speech disturbances were reported by Hyman[8] in 9% and 5% of the patients respectively.

Another interesting feature due to leukemic infiltration of the hypothalamus is pathologic weight gain, the hypothalamic syndrome. This was first described by Sansone in 1954 in two of 24 patients that he was treating for acute lymphocytic leukemia[13]. The pathological features of his two cases revealed parenchymal infiltration of the diencephalo-hypophyseal region and was manifested clinically by Frolich's obesity. Both of the patients responded to IT methotrexate. Shaw, in 1960[1], reported in his series a patient who had striking hyperphagia, pathologic weight gain, and behavioral disturbance and who at autopsy was found to have massive leukemic infiltration of the hypothalamus. He further collected about 12 cases from the literature from 1954-1960. Only five of the cases were on steroids at the time of the weight gain so steroids could not be implicated in all of the cases. In the present review, the incidence of abnormal weight gain was about 12%. Undoubtedly, some of these patients were on steroids so this figure may be an overestimation.

Ataxia was mentioned in two reviews and from these the overall incidence was determined to be $\simeq$ 6%. Ataxia in these patients may have been due to infiltration of the cerebellum. Hemiparesis was observed in three series for about a 6% incidence.

TABLE I
Symptoms
% of Patients in Which Symptoms Listed

Reference	# Pts.	N & V	Head-ache	Lethargy	Ocular dist.	Phychi. dist.
Shaw et al[1]	25	88%	56%	88%	44%	
Pierce[2]	26	92%				
Koch et al[3]	28	82%	68%	18%	4%	
Hardisty & Norman[4]	29	80%	70%		4%	
Haghbin & Zuelzer[5]	61	77%	84%		3%	
Nies et al[6]	27	13%	16%	28%		
Falkson et al[7]	12	23%	61%			
Hyman et al[8]	59	78%	76%	37%	40%	20%
Sullivan et al[9]	49	61%	63%	6%	22%	
Individual case reports[b]	39	36%	59%			
Average (%)		63%	61%	35%	20%	20%(1)[a]
# Pts from which average derived		357	331	190	253	59

a. (1) Indicates percentage derived from a single study
b. Derived from tables listed under therapy sections and denoted

TABLE II
Signs
% of Patients in Which Signs Listed

Reference	# Pts	Papill-edema	Suture Sep.	Facial Palsy	Periph Palsy	Pupil Change
Shaw et al[1]	25	64%	95%	36%		20%
Pierce et al[2]	26	96%		19%		
Koch et al[3]	28	39%	7%	25%	4%	
Hardisty & Norman[4]	29	70%		16%		
Haghbin & Zuelzer[5]	61			13%	5%	
Nies et al[6]	27	18%		14%		
Falkson et al[7]	12	23%		28%		
Hyman et al[8]	59	58%	51%	11%	7%	
Sullivan[9]	49	43%	18%	24%	6%	
Individual[b] case reports	39	31%	15%	15%		
Average (%)		49%	34%]	22%	5%	20%(1)[a]
# Pts from which average derived		296	229	357	199	25

a. (1) Indicates percentage derived from single study
b. Derived from tables listed under therapy sections and denoted by references

TABLE I
Symptoms
% of Patients in Which Symptoms Listed

Vertigo	Convul- sions	Coma	Abd. Pain	Irritability	Cheyne- Stokes Resp.	Aud. Dist.
	56%	44%				
	8%					
	21%	4%	7%	11%	4%	
	8%					
	5%					
	8%					
15%	8%	5%		14%	4%	9%
				37%		
	5%			20%		
15%(1)[a]	15%	17%	7%(1)[a]	20%	4%	9%
59	294	112	28	138	87	59

by references where 1-4 patients only were listed.

TABLE II
Signs
% of Patients in Which Signs Listed

Reflex Change	Ataxia	Hemi- paresis	Babinski's Sign	Wt Gain	Hydro- ceph	Abnormal EEG	Rigidity
40%			32%	4%		90%	28%
							46%
	11%	7%		11%	7%		4%
	4%			26%			
				8%			
							31%
		5%		14%	2%	75%	12%
	2%	2%		16%			18%
				5%		3%	18%
40%(1)[a]	6.0%	5.0%(1)[a]	32%(1)[a]	12%	7%(1)[a]	56%	22%
25	108	138	25	292	87	96	240

where 1-4 patients only are listed.

Electroencephalograms (EEG's) were done routinely in
only two studies. Shaw[1] reported that the incidence of abnormal EEG was 19 of the 21 patients. Two of the patients
could not be evaluated because they were receiving 6-azaur-
acil therapy. Of the remaining 19 patients, 17 had diffuse
dysrhythmias and two had focal abnormalities. The diffuse
patterns were non-specific theta and delta wave activity.
The focal changes were also non-specific. Hyman[8] reported
that 27 of 36 patients (75%) had abnormal EEG. In 20 of
the 27 there were diffuse dysrhythmias; eight of these had
slowing of the cycles. In the remaining seven, only a
portion of the brain appeared to be affected; the changes
included sporadic increased voltage, slowing of the cycles,
and disorganization in the bifrontal area.

Of the signs specific for meningeal irritation nuchal
rigidity was mentioned in about 22% of the cases. Specifically Kernig's or Brudzinski's signs were not mentioned.

The most consistent abnormality in patients with CNS
leukemia is the cerebrospinal fluid (CSF). The diagnosis
of leukemic meningiopathy is made when the presence of cells
are found in the CSF, and other clinical signs and symptoms
as described above are present. There are exceptions to
this; for in some patients, the meningeal signs and symptoms
may be present without CSF evidence of the disease; while
in others, the patient may be asymptomatic and have numerous
abnormal CSF findings. As can be seen from Table III, the
most commonly occurring abnormality in the CSF is increase
in the number of cells. Indeed the cells were increased in
$\simeq$ 89% of the patients with childhood ALL with an average
of the median cell count of $\simeq$ 530 cells/mm^3. In adults
with meningeal leukemia,in the 12 patients individually
reported, the cells were increased 100% of the time but
the median here was only 297 cells/mm^3. Why there would
be a difference and whether this difference is significant
is not known. Perhaps the number of cells is influenced
by age, or by the type of leukemia, since $\simeq$ 50% of the
adults in this series have AML.

In Hardisty and Norman's report[4], in most instances,
the cells were recognizable on stained smears as leukemic
blast cells, and mitotic figures were not infrequently seen.
There was no correlation between the initial CSF cell count
and the immediate response to treatment. However, a count
over 1000 cells per mm^3 was associated with an appreciably
higher incidence of early recurrence of meningeal involvement than that found after episodes in which the cell count
was below this figure. In Shaw's report[1], the cell counts
ranged from 26 to 11,000 per cubic millimeter. Examinations
of the fresh specimens under a phase microscope in many
instances permitted identification of the cells as abnormal,
leukemic blasts. No correclation existed between the CSF
white counts and the peripheral blood leukocyte counts.

TABLE III

Initial CSF Findings in Patients with CNS Leukemia

Reference	# Pts	% of Patients in Which Finding Abnormal				Med Values for Cerebrospinal Fluid Findings			
		Cells >10 per mm^3	Pressure >200mmH$_2$O	Sugar <50mg%	Protein >45mg%	Cells per mm^3	Pressure mm H$_2$O	Sugar mg%	Protein mg%
Shaw et al[1]	25	64%	89%	24%	16%				
Pierce[14]	26	100%	100%	41%	41%	167	375	50	23
Sullivan et al[9]	99			70%	48%	490	405		
Hyman et al[8]	59	84%	91%	55%	21%	547	335	38	34
Hardisty & Norman[4]	29	96%	66%		66%				
Rieselbach et al[15]	15						117		37
Individual Children[a] Case Reports	12-24	100%	75%	70%	50%	914	300	31	50
Individual Adults[b] Case Reports	7-12	100%	60%	43%	100%	297	230	50	74
Average of Children		89%	84%	52%	40%	530	306	40	35
Number of Pts from which Average Derived		139	139	209	238	184	199	85	100

a. Derived from tables listed under therapy sections and denoted by references where 1-4 patients only were treated.

b. Derived from table on treatment of adults with IT Methotrexate.

Routine bacteriologic cultures of the CSF were performed
on 18 patients and all were negative. Special cultures for
virus, fungi, and mycobacteria tuberculosis were done on
a number of other patients and these too were negative.
Hyman[8] did bacteriologic cultures on her patients in 64
episodes and all were negative. Indeed, she had not seen
a case of bacterial meningitis in any of the children
followed in her clinic although other types of infection
including septicemia did occur.

Approximately 11% of the patients did not evidence a
pleocytosis in the spinal fluid and their CNS leukemia was
diagnosed by symptoms and signs of meningeal leukemia.

There are also some patients who have CNS leukemia by
CSF evidence but do not manifest clinical symptomatology.
This would, of course, be expected from several large
autopsy series. For example, Leidler and Russell[16] concluded that ≃ 80% of leukemics have had significant pathological changes in the brain at necropsy indicating CNS
involvement but that only ≃ 20-35% of these patients
have neurologic symptoms or signs.

Two studies attempting to clinically determine, via
lumbar puncture, the presence of CNS leukemia in asymptomatic patients have been done. Evans et al[17], in 1963,
studied three groups of children in which 50 lumbar punctures were done in each group. The first group was composed
of symptomatic patients with CNS leukemia; the second group
was comprised of patients who had been treated for CNS
leukemia with methotrexate; the third group was composed
of leukemics without signs or symptoms of CSF involvement.
On Table IV, taken from the paper, is the data describing
the CSF findings in these three groups of patients.

As can be seen, the mean number of cells per mm^3 (620)
is in the symptomatic group close to the number derived from
various studies reported earlier. Also, in the treated
patients the cell counts normalize after IT methotrexate
(the therapy with methotrexate will be discussed in a later
section). What is most significant in reference to this
section is that the CSF findings in the asymptomatic patients who had counts slightly above normal (12, 18, and
37 cells/mm^3) but who failed to develop symptoms. The
authors concluded that the study indicated that the leukemic child who had never developed CNS manifestations
has a normal cerebrospinal fluid. In addition, the
CSF findings reflected the clinical symptoms, regardless
of when the lumbar puncture was done. Finally they stated
that "this good correlation between signs and cerebrospinal
fluid supports the belief that the CNS of the child who is
asymptomatic is uninvolved by the leukemic process"[17].

As derived from the methods used, these conclusions
are correct although they do refute the enormous patho-

TABLE IV
Cerebrospinal Fluid Findings in Children with Acute Leukemia[17]

CNS Status		Pressure (mmH$_2$O)	Cells (per mm^3)	Protein (mg/100 ml)	Sugar (mg/100 ml)	Blood Sugar (mg/100 ml)
Group I Symptomatic	Mean	394	620	42	40	92
	Range	(100–700+)	(18–3,400)	(5–220)	(<10–72)	(74–125)
Group II Following Treatment	Mean	300	17	30	55	86
	Range	(75–600)	(0–117)	(7–89)	(20–96)	(57–120)
Group III Asymptomatic	Mean	257	2	15	54	77
	Range	(100–440)	(0–37)	(7–60)	(30–90)	(45–120)

TABLE V
CSF Specimens[18]

Cell Count # of Cells/mm^3		# of Episodes	Cytological Findings			
			# of Episodes with Immature Cells 0	(%) of total Episodes	# of Episodes with Immature Cells 1 – 100	(%) of total Episodes
Within Normal Limits	0–4	227	135	(34.0%)	92	(23.4%)
	5–10	46	6	(1.5%)	40	(10.3%)
Definitely Abnormal	11–50	47	1	(0.5%)	46	(11.7%)
	>50	73	4	(1.0%)	69	(17.6%)
Total		393	146	(37.0%)	247	(63.0%)
# of Patients with Symptoms		103	26	(6.6%)	77	(19.6%)

logical data on patients with leukemia. Another study
which is in accordance with the pathological studies was
done by Nies et al[18] at the National Cancer Institute. They
studied a group of 78 leukemic patients randomly and took
a total of 393 CSF specimens. Not only were routine cell
counts and differentials done on the samples but in addition, cytology on millipore filtered fluid from the same
specimens was done. As can be seen from Table V, derived
from their data, there was a poor correlation between the
finding of abnormal cells on cytological examination and
the routine CSF count. Based on subsequent clinical data
and autopsy reports the incidence of definite false pos-
itives and negatives was only 4% and 6% respectively.

It becomes apparent that of the 273 episodes where
normal cell counts were found the cytology was abnormal
in 132 episodes(49%). Also, whereas abnormal cytology was
present in 63% of the episodes, only in 27% were signs or
symptoms present. Furthermore by obtaining clinical and
necropsy follow-up, the authors concluded that when the CSF
cytology was positive and the cell count normal, leukemia
infiltration of the arachnoid was likely in $\simeq$ 90% of
the patients with ALL (61 of 78 patients). Thus, abnormal
CSF cytology can be present in the leukemic patient who
is asymptomatic and who has a normal CSF count, and that
$\simeq$ 90% of such patients go on to develop CNS leukemia
either clinically or by necropsy. This study supports the
postmortem studies which found that CNS evidence of leukemia was present in $\simeq$ 80% of leukemics. These findings
speak loudly for prophylactic CNS therapy either in the
form of chemotherapy and/or radiotherapy in leukemia pa-
tiens with ALL.

Increased CSF pressure is the second most common abnormal CSF finding being present in $\simeq$ 84% of children
$\simeq$ 60% of adults in the studies reviewed. The median pressure was 306 mm of H_2O for children and 230 mm of H_2O in
adults. In Shaw's[1] series he reported two patients with
pressure elevations above 600 mm.

Perhaps the least reliable of the various characteristics of the CSF in patients with ML were the sugar and
protein values. The sugar was abnormally low (<50 mg/100 ml)
in 52% of the cases and the protein was abnormally high
(>40 mg/100 ml) in only 40% of the cases. This confirms the
belief of most investigators that the CSF protein values
are the least reliable indicators in the CSF of CNS leukemia. In the study by Pierce et al[28], he could find no
correlation between the low level of the spinal fluid
sugar and the cellular reaction. The low sugar cerebrospinal fluid sugar level has been attributed to increased
glyocolysis by the leukemic cells[1]. A decrease in the CSF
sugar level after _in vitro_ incubation with leukemia cells
has been described in two separate reports[1]. However,
Goldring and Hartford[19] suggest that alterations in the

"blood-brain barrier" may decrease the diffusion of glucose across this membrane and result in lower cerebrospinal fluid sugar levels.

In summary, of the CSF symptoms and signs, headache and increase in CSF cell count respectively are the most frequent manifestations of CNS leukemia. Abnormal CSF cytology may be present in the asymptomatic patient who has a normal CSF cell count. CSF protein and glucose values are less reliable than CSF cells and CSF pressure in determining presence of meningeal leukemia.

REFERENCES

1. Shaw, R.K., Moore, E.W., Freireich, E.J., and Thomas L.B. Meningeal leukemia. A syndrome resulting from increased intracranial pressure in patients with acute leukemia. Neurology 10: 823, 1960.

2. Pierce, M.I. Neurologic complications in acute leukemia in children. Pediat Clin N Amer 9: 425, 1962.

3. Koch, K., Reiquam, C.W., and Beatty, E.C., Jr. Acute childhood leukemia. Unusual complications. Rocky Mountain Med J 63: 50, 1966.

4. Hardisty, R.M., and Norman, P.M. Meningeal leukaemia Arch Dis Child 42: 411, 1967.

5. Haghbin, M., and Zuelzer, W.W. A long-term study of cerebrospinal leukemia. J Pediat 67: 23, 1965.

6. Nies, B.A., Thomas, L.B., and Freireich, E.J. Meningeal leukemia, a follow-up study. Cancer 18(5): 546, 1965.

7. Falkson, G., Van Eden, E.B., and Falkson, H.C. Meningeal leukaemia. Med Proc Johannesburg 15: 13, 1968.

8. Hyman, C.B., Bogle, J.M., Brubaker, C.A., Williams, K., and Hammond, D. Central nervous system involvement by leukemia in children. I. Relationship to systemic leukemia and description of clinical and laboratory manifestations. Blood 25: 1, 1965.

9. Sullivan, M.P., Vietti, T.J., Fernbach, D.J., Griffith, K.M., Haddy, T.B., and Watkins, W.L. Clinical investigations in the treatment of meningeal leukemia: radiation therapy regimens vs conventional intrathecal Methotrexate. Blood 34: 301, 1969.

10. Steffey, J.M. The central nervous system manifestations
    of leukemia. A report of 6 cases with meningeal involve-
    ment. J Pediat 60: 183, 1962.

11. Sullivan, M.P. Leukemic infiltration of meninges and
    spinal nerve roots. Pediatrics 32: 63, 1963.

12. Kanner, S.P., Wiernik, P.H., Serpick, A.A., and Walker,
    M.D., CNS leukemia mimicking multifocal leukoencephalo-
    pathy. Amer J Dis Child 119: 264, 1970.

13. Sansone, G. Pathomorphosis of acute infantile leukemia
    treated with modern therapeutic agents; "meningoleu-
    kemia" and "Frolich's Obesity". Ann Pediat (Basel)
    183: 33, 1954.

14. Pierce, M. Leukemia in children: treatment of 22 cases
    with 6-mercaptopurine. Ann N Y Acad Sci 60: 415
    1954.

15. Rieselbach, R.E., et al. Intrathecal aminopterin
    therapy of meningeal leukemia. Arch Intern Med 3:
    620, 1963.

16. Leidler, F., and Russell, W.O. The brain in leukemia.
    A clinico-pathologic study of twenty cases with a
    review of the literature. Arch Path 40: 14, 1945.

17. Evans, A.E. The cerebrospinal fluid of leukemic chil-
    dren without central nervous system manifestations.
    Pediatrics 31: 1024, 1963.

18. Nies, B.A., Malmgren, R.A., Chu, E.W. Del Vecchio, P.
    R., Thomas, L.B., and Freireich, E.J. Cerebrospinal
    fluid cytology in patients with acute leukemia. Cancer
    18: 1385, 1965.

19. Goldrin, S., and Harford, C.G. Effect of leucocytes
    and bacteria on glucose content of the cerebrospinal
    fluid in meningitis. Proc Soc Exp Biol Med 7: 669,
    1950.

III. Systemic Therapy for Meningeal Leukemia

A. General Considerations

1. Blood-Brain Barrier

For systemic chemotherapy to alter the course of meningeal leukemia, one must be able to deliver those drugs through the physiological barrier between the blood and the brain: the so-called "blood-brain barrier". Since the sanctuary of the leukemic cells also involves the CSF there are then three barriers that must be considered. These are the blood-brain barrier, the brain-CSF barrier and the blood-CSF barrier. As we have appreciated from the earlier chapter on pathology data in patients with meningeal involvement, it is necessary to traverse all three barriers since in many patients both CSF and parenchymal tissues are involved.

The actual location of these barriers is still the subject of intensive research but a few principles have evolved. The barrier between the blood and the brain appears to be the capillary endothelial cells in association with the tightly packed sheath of glial and neuronal cells which completely surrounds the brain capillary[1]. The blood-CSF barrier is predominantly composed of the secretory cells of the choroid plexus that secrete the spinal fluid. These cells form a barrier which separates a rich vascular supply from the pool of CSF. In addition, this barrier is not only passive but active; indeed, it has been shown to actively transport weakly ionized substances from the CSF to blood[2]. In this way, it has been compared to a "reverse renal tubule". Furthermore, the ependyma separates the CSF from brain parenchyma. Several studies have shown that these cells also may be responsible in part for secretion of spinal fluid. The ependymal cells are also involved in active secretion since both carbonic anhydrase inhibitors as well as dinitrophenol will partially inhibit this process[3].

Those characteristics which allow drugs to enter tissues in general are also acting to affect the entry of agents into the brain and CSF. These characteristics include small molecular size, high degree of lipid solubility, nonionization at physiological pH and lack of appreciable plasma protein binding[1]. The rate of exit of a drug from the CSF is also dependent in part on these characteristics but not entirely. This is because one must also include bulk flow as well as active transport and diffusion as a mechanism by which drugs leave the CSF.

Drugs may be included or excluded from the brain and CSF by one or all of the aforementioned mechanisms. Antipyrene for example, being a small molecule, lipid soluble, and nonionized enters the CSF rapidly and reaches a CSF-plasma concentration ratio of unity. Such ability to do this may be present in the nitrosourea group of anti-neoplastic agents since they also are lipid soluble, small, and nonionized molecules. For this reason, they are able to affect the course of meningeal leukemia both in animal systems and clinically (See chapter on BCNU treatment). Sulfadiazine, on the other hand, has a low degree of lipid solubility and is slightly ionized. Being of low lipid solubility, the drug enters the CSF very slowly[1]. Being slightly ionized, it can never reach unity between the blood and CSF, for the drug on the CSF side is non-ionized (due to lower pH) and is free to move out of the CSF once again and enter the blood[1].

The almost complete exclusion of compounds such as methotrexate or p-aminohippurate (PAH) can be explained by the fact that they are highly ionized and lipid insoluble at physiologic pH. Thus, they do not cross the blood-brain barrier well at all. Also, since after they enter, they tend to remain in the CSF pool exclusively, they can be removed quite rapidly by bulk flow mechanisms via the arachnoid villi and thus into the blood. It is now clear that some organic acids and bases are also actively trans-ported from the CSF. This is true for PAH, penicillin, as well as methotrexate. Thus whereas the CSF:plasma ratio of antipyrene is one, the CSF:plasma ratio of methotrexate is 0.05. The plasma binding of methotrexate by $\approx$ 50% also excludes a large amount from the CSF pool.

Drug exit from the CSF is by 3 mechanisms. These are active transport (primarily via the choroid plexus and ependymal cells), diffusion (primarily via the ependymal lining cells) and bulk flow (via the arachnoid villi). Thus, once a drug passes the blood-brain barrier, to be effective it must resist those forces which tend to remove it. Various methods have been attempted in preclinical systems to accomplish this goal. For example, one may use a competing drug such as PAH or probenecid to saturate the weak acid transport system from the CSF to blood and per-haps maintain higher levels of methotrexate in the CSF for longer periods of time. Changes in the acid-base balance of the animal may also have an effect by changing the ionization of compounds once in the CSF. For example, metabolic acidosis will increase the CSF:plasma ratio of sulfadiazine[1]. Finally by decreasing bulk flow (such as with carbonic anhydrase inhibitors), one would decrease this avenue of exit from the CSF.

The problem of the blood-brain barrier in the chemo-therapy of leukemia in general as well as meningeal leu-kemia is thus many faceted. It involves developing drugs which have as their characteristics properties which en-able them to enter the CSF and brain parenchyma. Once in,

methods should be developed which will enable those compounds to remain longer and in higher concentrations.

Since neither the ideal drug nor the ability to keep
drugs in the CSF has been developed, most chemotherapists
have resorted to intrathecal administration of agents such
as methotrexate in an attempt to eradicate meningeal
disease. However, as we shall see in the chapter on BCNU
therapy and pyrimethamine therapy, the goal of finding an
ideal drug for this purpose may be close at hand. Both
of these agents are small, nonionized, and lipid soluble
agents that have demonstrated clinical effectiveness in
the treatment of meningeal leukemia. Furthermore newer
nitrosoureas such as CCNU and Methyl-CCNU, both of which
are more lipid soluble than BCNU, may add further dimen-
sion to the treatment of CNS involvement by leukemia.

REFERENCES

1. Rall, D.P. Experimental studies of the blood-brain
    barrier. Cancer Res 25: 1572, 1965.

2. Broder, L.E., and Oppelt, W.W. Effect of benzolamide
    on cerebrospinal formation. Pharmacol Exp Ther 169:
    271, 1969.

3. Pollay, M., and Curl, F. Secretion of cerebrospinal
    fluid by the ventricular ependyma of the rabbit. Amer
    J Phys 213: 1031, 1967.

B. Miscellaneous Agents Used Systemically

There are several reports in the literature on the use of antileukemic drugs systemically in an effort to control CNS leukemia after its emergence. The reports are rather sporadic since radiotherapy and IT therapy became established at about the same time. The reports that do exist are summarized in Table I.

Poncher et al[1], in 1952, were the first to describe a child who developed signs of intracranial involvement while being treated with folic acid antagonists. Two months prior to his death he developed CNS leukemia.

Sansone[2], in 1954, reported the occurrence of meningeal leukemia in two patients treated with aminopterin and adrenal steroid hormones. The two patients with the longest survival developed this syndrome. The first patient was a boy age 9, with ALL, who went into complete remission following treatment with aminopterin. During the remission he developed headache, loss of muscle strength, visual defects, meningeal symptoms, paresthesias, and absence of the deep tendon reflexes. The spinal fluid showed the usual abnormalities associated with CNS leukemia with increased cells, protein, and decreased sugar concentrations. Retreatment

TABLE I
Meningeal Leukemia Treated Systemically

Reference	# Patients treated	Leukemia Type ALL	AML	Sex M	F	# Episodes	yrs. age	Hematol. CR	PR
Poncher et al, 1952[1]	1					1		1	
Sansone, 1954[2]	2	2			2	2	9,12	1	
Hamilton et al, 1954[3]	1				1	1	2		
Bernard et al, 1954[4]	1					1		1	
Sullivan, 1959[5]	1		1		1	1	3 1/2	1	
Shaw et al, 1960[6]	20					8 3 1 8	22 children 3 adults (total)		

with oral aminopterin was ineffective, because in the usual oral doses the drug does not cross the blood-brain barrier to a significant degree. Intrathecal aminopterin was then tried which resulted in moderate but transient clinical improvement and a marked reduction in the number of cells in the spinal fluid. The second patient reported by Sansone was a 12 year old boy with ALL, whose initial treatment with aminopterin and cortisone resulted in a complete remission. Four months after the initiation of treatment, he began gaining weight rapidly and developed meningeal signs. Spinal fluid was consistent with meningeal leukemia. The bone marrow at this time revealed complete relapse. The patient was retreated with aminopterin and cortisone with a resultant complete hematological remission but no change in the neurological symptoms. The patient was then given IT aminopterin for two doses with a resultant marked decrease in the spinal fluid cell count but little change in the clinical condition.

Hamilton and Elion[3] also noted the leukemic meningiopathy, in a girl of two, on whom studies of labelled 6-mercaptopurine (6-MP) were done. One month before the experimental studies were finished she developed objective and subjective findings of CNS leukemia. The patient was subsequently treated with 6-MP and azaserine without success. Bernard and Seligmann[4] in reporting 61 cases treated with 6-MP make special mention of their Case 40 in which "relapse was at first purely meningeal with high leukoblastosis in the CSF while the blood remained normal". "Treatment with 6-MP did not prevent progressive aggravation,

TABLE I

Meningeal Leukemia Treated Systemically

Status Rel.	Drug Dose	Objective Response CR	PR	NC	Subjective Response CR	PR	NC	Duration of CNS Remission after Rx.	Duration of Leukemia after Rx.	Survival
	Folic acid antagonists						1			22 mos.
1	Aminopterin and cortisone		2				2			12,16 mos.
1	6-MP and Azaserine		1				1			
	6-MP		1				1			
	6-MP and steroids		1				1			
	MTX			1			7			
	6-MP						3			
	MTX and 6-MP			1						
	Corticosteroids			5			3			

invasion of the blood and death[4]". It would appear that
in these patients the leukemia became resistant to 6-MP.
The mechanism of resistance to 6-MP has been proposed to be
due to a selection of cells deficient in an enzyme concerned
with the conversion of the analog to the corresponding
ribonucleotide. It is unlikely that the patients became resistant to the drug due to a blood-brain barrier block,
since this agent has been shown to cross the blood-brain
brain barrier sufficiently well[3].

Sullivan[5] reported in 1957 one case of meningeal leukemia in a 3 1/2 year old boy with AML. The patient went
into remission with methotrexate therapy but one month
later showed signs of increased intracranial pressure and
elevated protein in the spinal fluid. While on 6-MP maintenance, the patient developed signs and symptoms of CNS
leukemia unresponsive to 6-MP and adrenal steroids.

Shaw[6] reported on 25 patients with CNS leukemia treated
by various methods. He found that for the most part a
neurological improvement with systemic chemotherapy occurs
primarily when a systemic remission occurs. To evaluate
which drugs were effective in the management of meningeal
leukemia, only those compounds which had not been previously
administered to a patient were considered. Trial of antimetabolites given were methotrexate, 8; 6-MP, 3; and combination 6-MP and methotrexate,1; two (17%) of the 12 trials
resulted in an improvement in the meningeal leukemia, one
with MTX and one with combination therapy. Of the 8 trials
of corticosteroids, 5 resulted in both hematological remissions and sustained neurological improvement. Clinical
cures of meningeal leukemia were obtained with adrenal
steroids in two patients. The difference in the incidence
of CNS response to antimetabolites and steroids was not
statistically significant (P= 0.14).

As can be seen from Table I, the results of systemic
therapy have been relatively poor. The only agent which
shows much effect is corticosteroids. Out of a total of 26
patients, there have only been 7 responses (27%) with 5 of
these with adrenal steroids. As we shall see, this is less
than that seen with LP alone, IT therapy, BCNU therapy, or
radiotherapy.

REFERENCES

1. Poncher, H.B., Waisman, H.A., Richmond, J.B., Horak,
    O.A., and Limarzi, L.R. Treatment of acute leukemia
    in children with and without folic acid antagonists.
    J Pediat 41: 377, 1952.

2. Sansone, G. Pathomorphosis of acute infantile leukemia
    treated with modern therapeutic agents; "Meningoleukemia"
    and "Frolich's Obesity". Ann Pediat (Basel)183: 33, 1954.

3. Hamilton, L., and Elion, G.B. The fate of 6-mercap-
    topurine in man. Ann NY Acad Sci 60: 304, 1954.

4. Bernard, J., and Seligmann, M. A study of 61 leukemias
    treated with 6-mercaptopurine. Ann NY Acad Sci 60:
    385, 1954.

5. Sullivan, M.P. Intracranial complications of leukemia
    in children. Pediatrics 20: 757, 1957.

6. Shaw, R.K., Moore, E.W., Freireich, E.J., and Thomas,
    L.B. Meningeal leukemia. A syndrome resulting from
    increased intracranial pressure in patients with acute
    leukemia. Neurology 10: 823, 1960.

C. BCNU Therapy

BCNU will be considered separately as it is a unique compound in its ability to cross the blood-brain barrier. It is relatively unionized at physiological pH, and is quite lipid soluble. It, therefore, has those properties which permit easy passage across the blood-brain barrier.

1,3-Bis(2-chloroethyl)-1-nitrosourea (NSC-409962; BCNU) is one of the group of nitrosoureas having the empirical formula of $C_5H_9N_3O_2Cl_2$. It has the following structure:

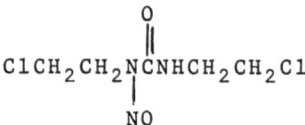

It has a molecular weight of 214.06, and 1 gram is soluble in $\simeq$ 250 ml of 0.9% saline solution, and 80 ml of propylene glycol. The Log P value, which is a measure of lipid solubility relative to water solubility of a nitrosourea compound, for BCNU is 1.39 for its distribution between decanol and water[1], making it quite lipid soluble.

The first step that led to the synthesis and demonstration of the marked experimental antileukemic activity of BCNU[2] was the notation of the weak activity of 1-methyl-3-nitro-1-nitrosoguanidine against IP L1210 in the CCNSC screen, and the demonstration of greater therapeutic activity for 1-methyl-1-nitrosourea and its clear-cut activity against IC L1210[3].

The biochemical effects of BCNU have been studied using several experimental techniques in various mouse, rat, hamster, and human tumor lines, cell free systems, microbiological studies, and by analytical chemistry. The oncolytic effect of the drug may be due to the inhibition of the synthesis of DNA and RNA. Observations related to the mechanism of action include: alkylation by formation of diazohydroxide and/or 2-chlorethylamine[4]; selective interference with the utilization of histidine in 1-carbon metabolism through the inhibition of formimino-transferase[5]; increase NADase activity and decreases the concentration of NAD+ in tumor cells[6]; decreases DNA nucleotidyltransferase activity[7].

Animal tumor data reveals (CCNSC Screening Data) that against intracerebral L1210 (IC) in mice, the percent 30 day day survivors were $\simeq$ 40% when $\simeq 10^5$ cells were inoculated and the drug was given IP at the LD_{10} dose.

Thomas[8] has shown BCNU capable of completely eradicating leukemic cells from both the extracranial organs and tissues and from the dural arachnoid and non-neural areas of the brain in mice inoculated IC with L1210 after institution of parenteral treatment with the drug. When L1210 is inoculated IC, parenteral BCNU kills 99% of intracerebral leukemic cells at the LD_{10} dose, as does cyclophosphamide, methotrexate, 6-MP, and 5-FU. However, at one-eighth of the LD_{10} dose, 90% of the cells are killed with BCNU as compared to 30-70% of the cells when the other drugs are used at this dose level. In mice inoculated IC (10^5 cells) or SC (10^5 - 10^6 cells) with L1210 leukemia and treated three days later with BCNU, the optimum dose was found to be 3.0 mg/kg/day. The median survival time was 34.5 days for treated IC tumors, 52.5 days for treated SC tumors, and 12 days for untreated controls.

Wodinsky and Kensler[9] has reported BCNU to be effective against intracranially implanted L1210 as well as leukemia L1798 and Dunning leukemia whereas cyclophosphamide was ineffective. Others have reported that in rats with IP or IC Dunning leukemia treated for 5 days with NSC-409962 there were a significant number of apparently tumor-free survivals noted.

In 1963, Rall reported giving BCNU to nine patients with ALL, five of whom had meningeal leukemia[10]. The dose range was 15-150 mg/m^2. No bone marrow remissions were seen in the leukemic patients but meningeal leukemia was controlled in all five patients. The predominant toxic effect was severe, prolonged bone marrow depression. Some increase in BUN and SGOT was seen. Pulmonary edema and pleural effusion occurred in three patients. Other toxic effects included dysphagia, esophagitis, anorexia and diarrhea. It was felt that the drug was uniquely effective when given orally in clearing meningeal leukemia.

Nies et al[11] in a follow-up study on meningeal leukemia reported the use of BCNU in three patients with far-advanced disease. In two children with ALL, BCNU was effective in reducing CSF cell count to normal. At autopsy neither patient had demonstrable leukemic infiltration of the arachnoid. In one patient with acute myelocytic leukemia (AML), treatment was not successful.

More recently, the Southwest Group[12] reported that IT methotrexate was superior to BCNU in maintaining CNS remissions in meningeal ALL when these CNS remissions were originally induced with methotrexate. In 46 evaluable patients 19 were treated with IT methotrexate, 14 were treated with BCNU, and 13 were given no treatment. The duration of CNS remissions were a mean of 488 days, 94 days, and 116 days respectively. They concluded that, "the superiority of the methotrexate regimen is of such degree that it should be considered for all children with CNS

TABLE I
Systemic BCNU in the Treatment of Meningeal Leukemia

Reference	# Patients treated	Leukemia Type		Sex	# Episodes	yrs. age	Hematol.		Status Rel.
		ALL	AML	M F			CR	PR	
Rall et al., 1963[10]	5	5			5	chil-dren			
Nies et al, 1965[11]	3	2	1		3	2 chil-dren 1 young adult			
Iriarte et al, 1966[13]	6	6		5 1	6	3-15 median 6	5		1
Sullivan et al, 1970[12]	46				19 14 13	children " "			

leukemia after remission is achieved". It thus appears that BCNU is inferior to IT methotrexate in maintaining remissions in CNS leukemia when original CNS remissions are induced with methotrexate. However, it does not answer the role that BCNU might play in inducing CNS remissions in the case where a CNS remission was originally induced with BCNU.

It is interesting to note that there may be cross resistance between BCNU and methotrexate when used in the treatment of meningeal leukemia. Iriarte, Hananian and Cortner have recently reported on the use of BCNU in 6 children with CNS leukemia[13]. The dose used was 150 mg/m^2 IV for three days. Three of the six children treated for CNS leukemia had a remission of their CNS manifestations. All three were experiencing first episode of CNS involvement by ALL and their marrows were in remission when BCNU was given. The three whose treatment failed had all had previous therapy for CNS involvement with either intrathecal methotrexate or radiation. Indeed, this may explain in part the results that Sullivan found above.

In summary then, BCNU has been used in about 14 children with 10 responses for an overall response rate of ≈ 71% (see Table I). Since the number of patients are so few it is difficult to compare the results with the other modes of therapy. Suffice it to say that it would appear that the response rate is similar to IT MTX. Significantly, for duration of remission, however, it is clearly inferior to MTX, after a MTX induced remission.

TABLE I

Systemic BCNU in the Treatment of Meningeal Leukemia

Drug Dose	Objective Response CR PR NC			Subjective Response CR PR NC			Duration of CNS Remission after Rx.	Duration of Leukemia after Rx.	Survival
15-150 mg/m² PO				5					
	2		1						2 mos. for the 2 children
150 mg/m² IV x3	3			3	3	3	4,7,22 mos.		
MTX 12 mg/m² q8wk IT							med. 16 mos.		
BCNU 100 mg/m² q8wk IV							med. 3 mos.		
No therapy							med. 3 1/2 mos.		

REFERENCES

1. A special report to Cancer Chemotherapy National Service Center. A summary of experimental data on nitrosoureas. Kettering-Meyer Laboratory, Southern Research Unit, December, 1969.

2. Johnston, T.P., McCaleb, G.S., and Montgomery, J.A. The synthesis of antineoplastic agents. XXXII. N-nitrosoureas. J Med Chem 6: 669, 1963.

3. Skipper, H.E., Schabel, F.M., Trader, M.W., and Thompson, J.R. Experimental evaluation of potential anticancer agents. VI. Anatomical distribution of leukemic cells and failure of chemotherapy. Cancer Res 21: 1154, 1964.

4. Wheeler, G.P., and Chumley, S. Alkylating activity of 1,3-bis(2-chloroethyl)-1-nitrosourea and related compounds. J Med Chem 10: 259, 1967.

5. D'Angelo, J.M., Groth, D.P., and Vogler, W.R. Effect of 1,3-bis(2-chloroethyl)-1-nitrosourea (BCNU) on purine metabolism. Int Cancer Congr Abstr 10: 408, 1970.

6. Green, S., and Bodansky, O. A relationship between NADase activity, NAD+ content and the proliferation of Ehrlich ascites cells. Proc Amer Assn Cancer Res 8: 23, 1967.

7. Wheeler, G.P., and Bowdon, B.J. Effects of 1,3-bis(2-
    chloroethyl)-1-nitrosourea and related compounds upon
    the synthesis of DNA by cell-free systems. Cancer Res
    28: 52, 1968.

8. Thomas, L.B. Pathology of leukemia in the brain and
    meninges. Cancer Res 25(9): 1555, 1965.

9. Wodinsky, I., and Kensler, C.J. Effectiveness of anti-
    tumor agents against intraperitoneally and intracere-
    brally inoculated Dunning leukemia in the Fischer rat.
    Nineth Int Cancer Congr Abstr 9: 380.

10. Rall, D.P., Ben, M., and McCarthy, D.M. BCNU toxicity
    and initial clinical trial. Proc Amer Assn Cancer Res
    4(1): 55, 1963.

11. Nies, B.A., Thomas, L.B., and Freireich, E.J. Meningeal
    leukemia, a follow-up study. Cancer 18(5): 546, 1965.

12. Sullivan, M.P., Haggard, M.E., Donaldson, M.H., and
    Krall, J. Comparison of the prologation of remission
    in meningeal leukemia with maintenance intrathecal
    methotrexate (IT MTX) and intravenous bis-nitrosourea
    (BCNU). Proc Amer Assn Cancer Res 11: 77, 1970.

13. Iriarte, P.V., Hananian, J., and Cortner, J.A.
    Central nervous system leukemia and solid tumors of
    childhood. Treatment with 1,3-bis-(2-chloroethyl)-1-
    nitrosourea (BCNU). Cancer 19: 1187, 1966.

D. CCNU

1-(2-chloroethyl)-3-cyclohexyl-1-nitrosourea (CCNU) is one of the group of nitrosoureas with the empirical formula of $C_9H_{16}ClN_3O_2$. It is lipid soluble and relatively unionized at physiological pH. Evidence points to the fact that it acts as a biologic alkylating agent but it may also, as shown with other nitrosoureas, inhibit several key enzymatic processes which ultimately lead to the formation of DNA. It was selected for clinical trial on the basis of its activity against mouse leukemia L1210. It is effective in daily treatment but more effective as a single treatment or when given in widely spaced treatment schedules (maximum ILS: >650%). Animal toxicology studies have revealed that the most dramatic and consistent toxicities involve the bone marrow, lymphoid tissue, liver, kidneys and gastrointestinal tract. Marrow depression occurred during the treatment period and was reversible if the animal survived the initial insult. Delayed liver damage was the principal dose-limiting toxicity, occurring as late as one month after the last dose and manifesting as elevated transaminase, alkaline phosphatase, and bromsulphalein values.

Clinically, the drug has finished a Phase I trial in various malignancies. Acutely, nausea and vomiting are seen while dose limiting delayed hematologic toxicity involving the platelets and leukocytes are seen at the maximum tolerated dose (MTD) of 130 mg/m^2 as a single oral dose. In contrast to the animal toxicologic data, there was no consistent hepatic or renal dysfunction during or after treatment with CCNU. At the MTD, responses have been observed in bronchogenic carcinoma, malignant lymphoma, and glioblastoma.

Used alone, responses have also been observed in gastrointestinal carcinoma (6/25), carcinoma of the breast (1/2) and carcinoma of the bladder (1/1). When used in combination with imidazole carboxamide and vincristine in malignant melanoma, 4/11 responses have been observed.

The drug is supplied in 40 mg and 100 mg capsules which when refrigerated at 4-10°C ensures the integrity of the dosage formulation for at least two years.

REFERENCES

1. Broder, L.E., and Carter, S.K. CCNU clinical brochure. National Cancer Institute, 1971.

E. Methyl CCNU

1-(2-chlorethyl-3-(4-methyl-cyclohexyl)-1-nitrosourea
(NSC-95441, Methyl-CCNU, Me-CCNU) is one of a group of
nitrosourea compounds developed by the Southern Research
Institute for the National Cancer Institute. Interestingly, this compound is the most lipid soluble of the
clinically useful nitrosourea compounds which include
BCNU and CCNU. The biochemical effects of the agent have
not been determined.

Me-CCNU is one the most active compounds screened
against a variety of solid tumor models in animals. This
is most apparent against the advanced Lewis lung tumor
where it cures mice when used alone and in surgical ad-
juvant tumor models. It is superior to both BCNU and CCNU
in this respect. It is also superior to these other nitrosoureas when used in early Lewis lung tumors, adenocar-
cinoma C3H of breast, and SC implanted melanoma B16.

Against the L1210 leukemia in mice, it is about midway
between BCNU and CCNU in effectiveness.

As with the other nitrosourea compounds, consistent
toxicities for Me-CCNU are seen in the bone marrow (hypo-
plasia), lymphoid tissue (atrophy and hemorrhage), liver
(altered liver enzymes), gastrointestinal tract (vomiting
and mucosal desquamation), renal (renal tubular damage) and
cardio-respiratory (edema, hemorrhage, myocardial infarct).
Quantitatively, BCNU and CCNU are more than twice as toxic
as Me-CCNU.

Pharmacolgical studies in the dog and monkey indicate
a quantitative difference in absorption of the drug orally
between the monkey and the dog. In the former, very little
of the agent is absorbed orally while in the latter, there
is very little difference in drug levels between oral and
IV administration.

The dosage formulation will be in 20, 50 and 100 mg
capsules which should be kept refrigerated at 4-10°C,
although normal room temperature storage for short periods
of time will not affect the potency of the drug.

REFERENCES

1. Broder, L.E., and Carter, S.K. Methyl CCNU brochure.
    National Cancer Istitute, 1971.

F. Pyrimethamine Therapy

Like BCNU, pyrimethamine, a 2,4-diaminopyrimidine, is another agent that has the ability to cross the blood-brain barrier. Those characteristics of lipid solubility and relative lack of ionization at physiological pH allow this compound relatively good access to the CNS when compared with methotrexate.

Pyrimethamine is a 2,4-diaminopyrimidine which was tested for and found to have antimicrobial activity in the early 1950's[1]. Pyrimethamine, the most active of this group of compounds has until recently been used exclusively for the prophylaxis and suppression of malaria in man[1]. Lately, in recognition of its action as a folic acid antagonist, it has been used in the therapy of neoplastic disease in polycythemia vera[2,3] and in the treatment of meningeal leukemia[4].

Pyrimethamine was originally developed from a series of drugs that exhibited the general property of antifolate activity in 1948[5]. That the drug was interfering with the reduction of folate was clear when folinic acid could overcome its effects in a bypass fashion both in bacteria and mammals[6]. As methotrexate, the drug has an affinity for and can inhibit dihydrofolate reductase with a K_i value of 1.8 x 10^{-6} for human liver enzyme[6]. This is $\simeq$ 900 times the K_i for methotrexate indicating a somewhat lower affinity for the enzyme than methotrexate. However, as was shown by Hitchings et al[6], the value for pyrimethamine was close enough to the K_m value for dihydrofolate (approximately 10^{-7}) that a high level of pyrimethamine could displace the substrate from the enzyme.

Differential toxicity between the host and intact microorganisms has been studied[1]. Apparently, dihydrofolate reductases from various sources exhibit difference in sensitivity to inhibition by pyrimethamine (Ferone et al, 1969). Thus, at doses that would be cytotoxic to protozoa, very little toxicity is seen in man. Indeed available evidence indicates that at doses of 25 mg per week no significant toxic symptoms have been reported for pyrimethamine[1]. When the drug was given at a dose of 25 mg/day in combination with sulisoxazole and prednisone (for the treatment of chorioretinitis[7]), megaloblastosis was produced. In short-term in vitro culture of the patient's bone marrow, the drug seemed to act as a folic acid antagonist producing defective deoxyuridine conversion to thymidylate. This was corrected poorly by oxidized and well by reduced folate. This concept of folinic acid rescue had been experimentally

TABLE I
Pyrimethamine in Meningeal Leukemia

Reference	# Patients treated	# Episodes	yrs. age	Hematol. CR	PR	Status Rel.
Geils[4]	1	2	36	2		

documented previously for pyrimethamine. Leucovorin could
be shown to alleviate the toxicity of the combination
pyrimethamine and sulfadiazine without interference with
chemotherapeutic effectiveness in the treatment of toxo-
plasmosis[6].

That pyrimethamine may cross the blood-brain barrier
has been demonstrated by its accumulation in the brain of
Rhesus monkeys[8], and in the case report of a patient treated for meningeal leukemia[4]. Schmidt et al[8] demonstrated
that drug accumulates in the brain of rats that had been
treated with daily oral doses of pyrimethamine for 42 days.
At all drug dosages the concentration in the cerebral
cortex was about 4 times the plasma and about twice the
muscle concentrations. Furthermore, at the higher doses of
drug, convulsions were produced.

Most recently, Geils et al[4] utilized the drug in the
therapy of meningeal leukemia (see Table I). The patient
was a 36 year old man who was found to have subleukemic
acute myeloblastic leukemia in 1964. A 6-MP and prednisone remission was successfully maintained with 25-50
mg of 6-MP daily for the subsequent 5 years. However,
in July of 1969, he developed symptoms and signs of meningeal leukemia. He was initially treated with methotrexate 0.2 mg/kg every other day for 4 treatments by subcutaneous reservoir technique. Due to development of
bacterial meningitis, this approach was discontinued.
Difficulty with lumbar puncture prompted the oral institution of pyrimethamine. He was given 75 mg daily for
4 days then 100 mg daily. After 5 days of pyrimethamine
therapy, the patient improved dramatically symptomatically.
After 11 days of therapy, the spinal fluid contained only
two blasts from an initial 156. Symptomatic thrombocytopenia necessitated termination of pyrimethamine therapy
and administration of folinic acid after 26 days of
therapy.

The first CNS remission lasted 7 months. A subsequent
CNS relapse (February 1970) was again treated with pyrimethamine with equally good results, lasting another 6

TABLE I

Pyrimethamine in Meningeal Leukemia

Drug Dose	Objective Response CR PR NC	Subjective Response CR PR NC	Duration of CNS Remission after Rx.	Duration of Leukemia after Rx.	Survival
75-150 mg PO daily then 25 mg daily maintenance	2		7 mos. 9 mos.	11 mos. after second episode	6 yrs.

months. The patient died in December 1970 with systemic relapse.

Spinal fluid analyses for pyrimethamine were done and revealed the drug level in the CSF ≃ 10-25% of the corresponding plasma level. (No evidence of accumulation of the drug in the spinal fluid after repeated dose was found.)

An important difference between methotrexate and pyrimethamine was illustrated by this case. Methotrexate, being relatively lipid insoluble and ionized a physiological pH, does not cross the blood-brain barrier in therapuetic amounts when given in tolerable oral or parenteral doses[9]. Pyrimethamine, which is lipid soluble and nonionized[10], has the ability to cross the blood-brain barrier as was demonstrated in Geils' et al paper. There appears to be a critical plasma level of the drug below which very little drug enters the CSF. In view of this, a different dosage schedule utilizing a large single dose rather than divided doses was suggested by the authors as being possibly more advantageous.

REFERENCES

1. Goodman, L.S. and Gilman, A. The pharmacological basis of therapeutics. New York, the Macmillan Co., 1970.

2. Isaacs, R. Treatment of polycythemia vera with Daraprim JAMA 156: 1491, 1954.

3. Israëls, M.C.G. Treatment and prognosis of polycythaemia managed by non-radioactive methods. Proc Roy Soc Med 59: 1100, 1966.

4. Geils, G.F., Scott, C.W., Baugh, C.M., and Butterworth, C.E., Jr. Treatment of meningeal leukemia with pyrimethamine. Blood 38: 131, 1971.

5. Hitchings, G.H., Elion, G.B., VanderWerff, H., and Falco, E.A. Pyrimidine derivatives as antagonists of pteroylglutamic acid. J Biol Chem 174: 765, 1948.

6. Hitchings, G.H., Burchall, J.J., and Ferone, R. Letters to the editor. New Eng J Med 281: 564, 1969.

7. Waxman, S. and Herbert, V. Mechanism of pyrimethamine-induced megaloblastosis in human bone marrow. New Eng J Med 280: 1316, 1969.

8. Schmidt, L., II., Hughes, H.B., and Schmidt, I.B. The pharmacological properties of 2,4-diamino-5-p-chloro-phenyl-6-ethyl-pyrimidine (Daraprim). J Pharmacol Exp Ther 107: 92, 1953.

9. Whiteside, J.A., Philips, F.S., Dargeon, H.W., and Burchenal, J.H. Intrathecal amethopterin in neurological manifestations of leukemia. Arch Intern Med 101: 279, 1958.

10. Hitchings, G.H. Discussion of paper (by Bertino et al.). Fed Proc 28: 896, 1967.

IV. INTRATHECAL THERAPY

A. Lumbar Puncture (LP)

When evaluating the results seen in the treatment of meningeal leukemia by the various methods of IT chemotherapy, one must pay heed to a control group of patients, those that have only received LP alone. These patients represent palliative placebo effect of IT therapy, similar in a sense to that which is measured when a drug is being evaluated for effect systemically. Thus, when evaluating the results of various investigators who have listed their responses in terms of only symptomatic response, the palliative effect could play a significant role in terms of response rate. This should be kept in mind in evaluating the response data in the following sections. There are at least three excellent papers in which this palliative effect of LP alone was measured.

D'Angio[1], in 1959, reported on the comparison between LP alone, LP plus radiotherapy, and radiotherapy alone. Twenty-four episodes received only radiotherapy and 62 episodes were treated with only LP (38 of these patients subsequently were given radiotherapy). It was of considerable interest that the condition of about 1/2 of the patients (42%) improved after lumbar puncture alone (See Table II). Although the actual mechanism by which relief is obtained is not known, they postulated that possibly the removal of fluid, together with any extradural leakage which may occur, is sufficient to relieve the pressure and restore the normal dynamics. The average interval of relief following lumbar puncture alone was one month except for an unusually long response of 15 months in one patient.

Roentgen therapy, with or without prior lumbar puncture, produced the greatest degree of lasting benefit as 75% of children were so helped. Following roentgen therapy alone, the average period before recurrence was three months;

TABLE I
Comparison of Three Modes of Therapy for ML[2]

	Lumbar Puncture Alone	Radiotherapy	Intrathecal Methotrexate
Number of episodes	50	50	50
Number of successfully treated patients	24 (48%)	49 (98%)	44 (88%)
Symptom-free interval			
Mean (in months)	0.6	2.8	3.7
Range (in months)	0 to 5	0 to 10	0 to 19

TABLE II
Meningeal Leukemia Treated by Lumbar Puncture Alone

Reference	# Pts.	Leukemia type ALL	AML	Sex M F	# episodes	yrs. age	Hematol. Status CR	PR	Rel.
D'Angio et al, 1959[1]	37	37		20 27	62	children av. 5 1/2			
Evans et al, 1964[2]	53				50	children			
Hyman et al, 1965[3]					43	children			

while following combined lumbar puncture and roentgen therapy, it was four months. Thus, one could employ duration of response as another means by which the results of therapy can be determined.

Evans[2], in 1964, compared three different modes of therapy. One was simple LP, one IT methotrexate, and the other radiotherapy. About 2-5 ml of CSF were removed. Fifty-three patients were studied who had 150 episodes of meningeal leukemia. Fifty episodes were accumulated for each treatment group. The results of the therapy are summarized in Tables I & II.

As can be seen again, ≃ 50% of the patients responded symptomatically to LP, while about twice as many responses were seen in the IT methotrexate group and the radiotherapy group. This could be interpreted as a 50% placebo effect. As will be seen in the next section, there is good correlation between the objective and subjective response rates with IT methotrexate. The duration of symptomatic relief following the LP only treatment was less than one month; while for the IT therapy and radiotherapy, the symptom free interval was about 2-3 months.

Hyman et al[3], in 1965, studied 36 patients with ALL in which there were 43 episodes of meningeal leukemia (See Table II). All patients initially received LP and their responses were evaluated. About 4-8 ml of fluid were removed with each LP. Symptomatic responses were seen in 19 out of the 43 or for a 44% response rate. Subsequent lumbar punctures were done and within two days the results of the CSF parameters were followed. As would be expected the CSF was lowered from a median of 360 mm H_2O on the first LP to a median of 310 mm H_2O at the second LP. However, the cells increased from median of 319 cells/mm^3 on the first puncture to 376 cells/mm^3 on the second, and both the CSF protein and sugar increased slightly (by 8 and 5 mg% respectively). Thus, except for decreasing the CSF pressure, the other parameters of objective CSF response were not seen. This data supports the view of

TABLE II

Meningeal Leukemia Treated by Lumbar Puncture Alone

IT Dose	Objective Response CR PR NC	Subjective Response CR PR NC	Duration of CNS Remission after Rx.	Duration of Leukemia after Rx.	Survival
		26	1 mo.		
		24	0.6 mos.		
		19			

D'Angio[1] that one reason for the decrease in symptomatology could be due to a lowering of the CSF pressure. The duration of remission by the very design of the study (with repeat LP done in two days) could not be determined. All the patients were then subsequently started on methotrexate. IT methotrexate in this same group of patients achieved an 85% symptomatic response rate and a 90% objective response rate. In this study, as in all the others, the objective and subjective responses to IT methotrexate correlated quite well.

REFERENCES

1. D'Angio, G.J., Evans, A.E., and Mitus, A. Roentgen therapy of certain complications of acute leukemia in childhood. Amer J Roentgen 82: 541, 1959.

2. Evans, A.E., D'Angio, G.J., and Mitus, A. Central nervous system complications of children with acute leukemia. An evaluation of treatment methods. J Pediat 64: 94, 1964.

3. Hyman, C.B., Bogle, J.M., Brubaker, C.A., Williams, K., and Hammond, D. Central nervous system involvement by leukemia in children. II. Therapy with intrathecal methotrexate. Blood 25: 13, 1965.

B. Folic Acid Antagonists

1. Methotrexate

Six years after Farber's[1] et al first description of
the systemic use of antifolic agents in patients with ALL,
Sansone[2] first described their use intrathecally in meningeal leukemia. In both instances, these two events have
been milestones in the treatment of patients with acute
leukemia. The use of methotrexate in both methods are
still mainstays in the attempt to eradicate the last leukemic cell.

The basis for the use of methotrexate lies in the fact
that antifolic agents such as amethopterin (methotrexate,
MTX) or aminopterin competitively inhibits the enzyme
dihydrofolate reductase, thus restricting the availability
of tetrahydrofolic acid to cells[3,4]. More specifically, the
enzyme blocks the conversion of folate to dihydrofolate
and tetrahydrofolic acid (THF) thereby critically limiting
the metabolic transfer of one-carbon units in a variety of
biochemical reactions. Those reactions, which are of special
importance in cellular reproduction, are the biosynthesis
of thymidylic acid, the nucleotide specific to DNA, and
inosinic acid, the precursor of adenine and guaninine
nucleotides in de novo purine biosynthesis. In human leukocytes, the synthesis of DNA appears to be more sensitive
than that of RNA to inhibition by methotrexate, suggesting
the most important effect of the drug is on thymidylate
synthesis.

In animals the mechanism of resistance to the drug has
been carefully investigated[5]. A common mechanism of resistance to methotrexate occurs through the development of
increased dihydrofolate reductase activity[6,7], and it appears
that in resistant cells the rate of enzyme synthesis may
exceed the rate of methotrexate uptake[8]. The rate of
methotrexate uptake by cells has been in itself shown to
correlate with the drug's ability to prolong the life of
tumor-bearing mouse hosts[9].

The problem of drug resistance has been studied in
great detail by Welch[10] and other investigators. Nichol[11,12,13]
studied the relative capacity of methotrexate to inhibit
dihydrofolate reductase in vitro. In much of his work, cells
of methotrexate-sensitive and resistant strains of line
I leukemia were used. The difference in the susceptibility
of the enzyme system to the inhibitory effects of the drug
with the two types of intact cells was quite small on the
order of four-fold. However, it was appreciated that this
degree of alteration in biochemical susceptibility to
MTX is quite sufficient to account for the resistance to
the drug which had been observed in vivo. However, sub-

sequent studies[14] utilizing the L1210 mouse leukemia system demonstrated that the development of drug resistance
in vivo, at least in the treatment of single animals with
methotrexate, was not responsible for the death of the
animals. Law found in a methotrexate-sensitive leukemia
(L1210), treated with methotrexate, that even though the
survival time of the treated animals was approximately
doubled as compared to that of untreated controls, leukemia
cells obtained from the treated mice just before death,
and inoculated into new animals, were still quite suscep-
tible to methotrexate.[14] Similar experiments were done by
Jaffe and Sweedler[10]. They determined the growth rate of
methotrexate sensitive cells in the peritoneal cavity of
mice both in methotrexate treated animals and untreated
controls. It was found that the untreated controls died
≈ 6 days following inoculation with tumor cells, and had
≈ 800 million such cells in the peritoneal cavity just
before death. The treated animals lived ≈ 12 days but just
before death had only 200 million viable cells in the
peritoneal cavity. By following the daily curve of the
number of tumor cells in the peritoneal cavity and by
noticing that after each treatment with methotrexate every
48 hours the number of viable cells would decrease significantly, they reasoned that the cells maintained their
sensitivity to methotrexate. Indeed, by transfering those
cells to other mice and continuing to treat them with
methotrexate, they found that only after four-successive
passages through drug treated mice, a strain of cells was
obtained which caused fatal leukemia unaffected by the
usual doses of methotrexate (a methotrexate resistant
strain of cells). Thus, the cells, found in the peritoneal
cavity at the time of death of methotrexate treated animals
with L1210 leukemia (IP), were still sensitive to methotrexate.

Since the drug had significantly decreased the number
of tumor cells in the peritoneum and the cells were still
sensitive to methotrexate, the question was raised by
Welch[10] in his review as to why those animals had died.
He reasoned that since the cells were still sensitive to
methotrexate the problem was not one of resistance. He
further postulated that perhaps the mice were dying due
to effects of leukemia cells growing elsewhere than in the
peritoneal cavity in sanctuaries that would not be reached
by methotrexate, such as the CNS.

Since methotrexate is highly ionized and water soluble,
it would not be expected to cross the blood-brain barrier
and this is indeed so. This was confirmed in man by
Whiteside et al[15] who studied the drug concentrations of
methotrexate in the blood and CSF after the drug was either
given by mouth or IT. By mouth, 0.33 mg/kg of methotrexate
gave a peak serum level of 900 γ/ml at 30 minutes which
dropped precipitously after three hours, while the CSF
drug level achieved a peak of only 15 γ/ml, after three

hours. However when the drug was given IT at 0.1 mg/kg, the peak levels were 300 times greater, in the CSF achieving 5000 γ/ml at one hour and was present at 30 times the level reached by the oral route at 18 hours. Interestingly, the five patients so treated had meningeal leukemia which was "resistant" to orally administered methotrexate but responded in all five cases to IT drug. The remissions obtained were probably attributable to the higher concentrations of drug at the site of lymphoblastic growth which resulted in cytolysis of the malignant cells which were previously quite resistant to the concentrations attainable by transport across the blood-brain barrier.

Recognition of these concepts may have prompted Sansone to attempt intrathecal therapy with aminopterin in 1954[2]. Two of his patients were not responding to conventional oral aminopterin. He, therefore, attempted the use of the same compound intrathecally. Aminopterin is an analog of methotrexate that differs structurally from that compound only by the substitution of a hydrogen instead of a methyl group on the N^{10} nitrogen. However, this substitution confers on the compound a 5-10 times increase in the antifolic activity. In one patient, he used 0.036 mg IT x 6 days and in the second case 0.025 mg IT x 2 days every other day. In both cases, there was a marked decrease in the cell count toward normal. Clinically, one of the patients improved while the other showed no improvement in the general condition.

It was 5 years after this first use of IT antifolics that additional investigators began reporting their results. In 1959, several reports on the use of IT methotrexate were published. Hyman et al[16] reported the use of methotrexate in nine children with acute leukemia who had CNS manifestations. They received 0.2 mg/kg during a 6-12 day period. Symptomatic improvement began in 8 instances 2-10 days after the first injection; in one it began immediately following the diagnostic puncture. In four instances, complete symptomatic remissions were obtained lasting 71, 78, 125, and 140 days. In four other instances, partial symptomatic relief was obtained lasting 8, 27, 38, and 60 days. Spinal fluid counts showed a decrease in 7 of the cases within 2-6 days and were normal in 6-28 days. The impression of the authors was that IT methotrexate had at least the same therapeutic effect as radiotherapy in the treatment of meningeal leukemia.

Cramblett[17], also in 1959, reported on four cases of meningeal leukemia treated with IT methotrexate. In those four cases, there were 7 episodes treated. All but one episode responded to the therapy, and in that episode, the peripheral disease caused death before the effects of therapy could be realized. In all cases that responded, the cells and other spinal fluid modalities normalized from two to four weeks. Murphy[18], in a review that same

year, described the results of treatment in 23 patients
who he grouped according to either objective signs with
increased intracranial pressure or subjective symptoms
with weakness of the lower extremities. Twelve of fourteen
patients with increased intracranial pressure had a good
response to IT therapy with methotrexate, while none of
the patients with weakness of the lower extremities responded. Perhaps those patients with weakness of the lower
extremities had far advanced disease.

In the same year, Whiteside et al[15], reported on the
treatment of five patients with neurological symptoms due
to leukemia and lymphosarcoma. The symptoms improved markedly with methotrexate at a dose of 0.1 to 0.5 mg per kg
IT. The neurological remissions began about one week after
instillation and lasted about 6 weeks. Repeated neurological
remissions were obtained in all patients. Two of the patients
were considered refractory to the drug orally, yet they
responded to the drug IT. The authors based this type of
response on the higher CSF levels of the drug which could
be obtained when given IT, as they showed by pharmacologic
studies on several of the patients. As they had previously
demonstrated in dogs, IT methotrexate produced a megaloblastosis in the bone marrow. A single dose of 1.8 mg/kg
in the dog caused death from marrow depression and damage
to the gastrointestinal epithelium. Repeated doses of the
drug were given to the patients with no ill effects. They
felt that the use of IT methotrexate would become a useful
tool in the armamentarium of the clinician treating acute
leukemia.

That he was right is evidenced by the more than 25
papers reporting individual case reports or larger series
numbering as many as 100 patients in which the drug was
used IT for meningeal leukemia. In this review, the results
of these various investigators will be discussed and compared with other treatment modalities including radiotherapy,
combined radiotherapy and chemotherapy and the use of drugs
other than IT methotrexate. The results of individual
investigators which until now have been considered separately will be included in the overall analysis. Table I
lists the various investigators and the results obtained
in children with meningeal leukemia.

From the data presented it becomes apparent that some
investigators analyzed only subjective responses, some only
objective responses, while others listed responses in both.
categories. Generally, the subjective response agreed quite
well with the objective responses. Table II summarizes the
results in Table I.

It can be appreciated therefore, that the order of overall response rate in meningeal leukemia treated with IT
methotrexate alone is of the order of 80-83%. To be able
to determine whether this response rate is significantly

TABLE I
Intrathecal Methotrexate in Meningeal Leukemia of Children

Reference	# patients	Leukemia Type ALL	AML	Sex M	F	# episodes	yrs. age	Hematol. Status CR	PR	Rel.
Hyman, C.B. et al, 1959[16]	9					10	2-12			
Whiteside et al, 1959[15]	5					5	children			
Cramblett, H.G., 1959[17]	4	4		3	1	7	1-5	3		1
Murphy, M.L., 1959[18]	23	23				23	children			
Shaw, R.K. et al, 1960[19]	4					4	children			
Laurance, B.M., 1961[20]	2	1	1	1	1	3	3,7 1/2			2
Zimmerman, V.H., 1961[21]	1	1		1		1				
Cottom, D.G.[22]	1	1		1		2	4 3/4	1		
Pierce, M.I., 1962[23]	15					15	av:4	6		9
Steffy, J.M., 1962[24]	5	4 (blast	1 CML)	3	2	8	3-5	2		3
Wegelius, R. et al, 1963[25]	2		2	1	1	2	2,4			2
Evans, A.E. et al, 1963[26]	53					50	children			
Hyman, C.B., et al, 1965[16]	36					67	3 mos.-13 yrs.			
Haghbin, M. & Zuelzer, 1965[27]	61			39	22	58	children			
Yakar, D. & Padeh, B., 1966[28]	1	1	1			1	19	1		
Koch, K. et al, 1966[29]	28					19/44	children			
Hardisty, R.M.& Norman, 1967[30]	29	29		14	15	42	children	24		26
Peter, A. et al, 1967[31]	1	1		1		1	3			1
Falkson, G. & Van Eden, 1968[32]	10	12		8	4	13	5-20	6		4
Selawry, O.S. & Odom, 1968[32]	26	26				26	children	26		
Sullivan, M.P. et al, 1969[34]	51					51	children			
Sullivan, M.P. et al, 1965[35]	102					102	children			
Kanner, et al, 1970[36]	1	1				1	4	1		

TABLE I
Intrathecal Methotrexate in Meningeal Leukemia of Children

IT Dose	Objective Response CR	PR	NC	Subjective Response CR	PR	NC	Duration of CNS Remission after Rx.	Duration of Leukemia after Rx.	Survival
0.2 mg/kg x 3-5	7		3	4	4	2	med. 2 mos.		
0.1-0.5 mg/kg					5		1-1 1/2 mos.		
2.5-5.0 mg x 1-3	6		1	6		1		5,6 mos. in 2	
0.2-0.5 mg/kg x 3		12	2			9	med. 5 mos.		
0.2-04 mg/kg	3		1	3		1	1-1 1/2 mos.		
10 mg x 2-3	2	1		2		1		7,8 mos.	18,22 mos.
	1			1					
5 mg x 3	2			2			>1 month		
0.2-0.4 mg/kg				5	3	7		med.5 1/2 mos.	for hem rem
1.0-5.0 mg x 1-3	8			2		1		6,12,16 mos.	24,28,29,32 mos.
0.5 mg x 4	2							3 mos.	
0.5 mg/kg x 1-2				44		6	med. 3.7 mos.		
0.2 mg/kg x 4				43	14	10	med. 2.5 mos.		
0.1 mg/kg							med. 5.4 mos.		
10 mg x 3	1			1					
				14	4	1			17.1 mos. mean
5-10 mg				42					18.0 mos. med
5 mg x 3	1			1					
0.5 mg/kg x 4	13			13				med. 3.4 mos.	
12 mg/m^2 x 2-6	26						see text		
2.0 mg/kg TD	40		11	37		14	med. 3 mos.		
12 mg/m^2 BIW	83	19							
10 mg/m^2 x 6	1			1			> 1 yr.		

TABLE II
Intrathecal Methotrexate

	# Pts.	# Episodes	Objective			Subjective		
			CR	PR	NC	CR	PR	NC
Evaluated Objectively (CSF)	144	144	111	12	21			
Evaluated Subjectively (Symptoms and Signs)	178	212				153	26	33
Evaluated by both criteria	88	97	80	1	16	69	8	20
% of Episodes			75%	5%	20%	72%	11%	17%
Overall Response Rate				80%			83%	
Combined Response Rate					81.5%			

different from other treatment modalities that include
methotrexate (such as IT methotrexate and radiotherapy)
would be quite difficult and would require the analysis
of a large number of patients in large comparative studies.
Several individual investigators, however, have asked this
very question in several papers and have attempted to
determine whether combinations of therapy are any better
than IT methotrexate alone. These studies will be discussed
in a subsequent section.

The response to IT methotrexate is often dramatic and
can be appreciated usually within the first week of therapy
as both amelioration of symptoms and signs and as a decrease
in the CSF cell count toward normal. Usually if the patient
responds both objective and subjective criteria are normalized in ≃ 2-4 weeks. As can be seen from Table I, most
investigators either measured response as survival after
meningeal complications or a duration of the CSF remission.
Some papers only gave overall survival of the group of patients with meningeal leukemia. The range of CNS remission
duration varied from about one month in some series to
≃ 5.4 months in others with the median duration of CNS
remission being ≃ 3 months. The duration of leukemia following therapy for meningeal leukemia ranged between 0.5 months
and 18 months with the median being ≃ 6 months. As was discussed previously, the patients with meningeal leukemia are
a selected group of patients which, by nature of their
longer survival, tend to develop meningeal leukemia. In all
of the papers in which the survival of the patients was
given, the patients lived at least 1.5 years.

Selawry and Odom[33] reported an interesting finding in
a group of patients they treated for meningeal leukemia.
In their study, they found the median duration of remission to be ≃ 4 months in 106 of 222 children with ALL, who
developed leukemia meningopathy and received IT methotrexate
alone or combined with radiotherapy. They further tested
about 26 patients in which 22 received either weekly or
bi-weekly methotrexate at a dose of 12 mg/m^2 for 2-3 doses.
Normalization of the CSF occurred within 14 and 9 days
respectively for the two schedules of methotrexate, with
the duration of remission being 143 days and 133 days respectively. However, four additional patients received methotrexate bi-weekly for ≈5-6 doses and their duration
of remission increased to a median of 225+ days. They
concluded that at least 8 or more IT doses of methotrexate
are necessary to approach eradication of leukemia meningopathy. These figures were based on the average number of
leukemic cells in the CSF space to be ≃ 10^8 at the time
of abnormal findings and the median cell kill per dose of
methotrexate to be ≃ 10^1 cells.

Up to now we have been discussing primarily children
with ALL. In several of the reports listed on the Table I,

TABLE III
Intrathecal Methotrexate in Meningeal Leukemia of Adults

Reference	# Patients	Sex M.	Sex F.	Leuk. Type	# Episodes	age yrs.	Hematol. Status CR.	PR	Rel.
Shaw et al, 1960[19]	3	2	1	2 ALL	2				
				1 AML	1				
Shanbrom et al, 1961[38]	2	2		1 ALL	3	25	1		
				1 AML	1	26			1
Baker, G.P. et al, 1962[39]	1	1		1 AML	1	28	1		
Soscia, J.L. et al, 1964[40]	1	1		1 ALL	2	25	1		
Spiers, A.S. et al, 1966[41]	1	1		1 ALL	2	48	1		
MacDougall, 1964[42]	1	1		1 AML	1	56	1		
Baike, A.G., 1967[43]	1		1	1 AML	1	52	1		
Suh, K.S., 1967[44]	1	1		1 ALL	3	32	1		
Kwaan, H.C. et al, 1969[45]	1	1		1 CGL to AML	2	55			1
Falkson et al, 1968[32]	1	2		1 ALL	2	38			1
	1			1 ALL	2	29	1		
Oldstone et al 1968[46]	1	3		1 ALL	1	50			
	1			1 AML	1	29			
	1			1 CGL to ALL	1	36			

a few of the cases were children with AML. There was no
mention of differing responses between AML and ALL. Specifically, Laurance[20] in his study had one patient with AML
and CNS complications who responded quite well to IT
methotrexate. Steffey[24] described one patient with CGL who
had a two month remission following IT methotrexate. In a
report by Nies[37] utilizing IT aminopterin, four of the
patients had AML and all responded to therapy. Several of
the larger series also included children with AML but did
not mention specifically any difference in response rate.

In the adults with meningeal leukemia, the incidence
of AML is higher. If a difference in response existed, it
should be apparent here. However, due to the lower incidence of meningeal leukemia in adults, only 7 cases of AML
in adults with meningeal leukemia have been reported out
of a total experience of 17 patients. Those investigators'
reports are listed on Table III.

As can be seen, the ages ranged from 25 years old
to 55 years old. In most cases, the patients were or had

TABLE III

Intrathecal Methotrexate in Meningeal Leukemia of Adults

IT Dose	Objective Response CR	PR	NC	Subjective Response CR	PR	NC	Duration of CNS Remission After Rx.	Duration of Leukemia After Rx.	Survival
0.2-0.4 mg/kg									
5-10 mg x 3	3			3				2 years	2 1/2 yrs.
5-10 mg x 3		1			1			2 mos.	3 mos.
10-20 mg x 3 to 135 mg TD				1			4 mos.	4 mos.	2 1/4 yrs.
20.0mg x 3	1				1				
15 mg x 2 and X-RT	1			1			1 mo.	3 mos.	13 mos.
75 mg TD	1			1			10 mos.		13 mos.
15 mg x 3	1			1			6 mos.	10 1/2 mos.	alive
15 mg x 2				1			4 mos.	4 mos.	alive
10-35 mg x 6 and X-RT	1			1			3 mos.	3 1/2 mos.	4 mos.
up to 12 mg/m^2	1			1					
up to 12 mg/m^2	1			1					
40 mg TD	1			1					
50 mg TD	1			1					
28 mg TD	1			1					

been on some type of antileukemic agent before the onset of meningeal leukemia. Of the adults listed in Shaw's[19] series, two had ALL and one had AML. It is not however, mentioned in that report if the adults definitely received methotrexate or not and therefore cannot be included in the overall response rate. This then leaves us with ≃ 14 patients which can be evaluated for response. Of these 14 patients, 8 were in remission, 3 in relapse, and in 3, the hematological status was not given. All of the patients received methotrexate in divided doses ranging from ≃ 2.5 mg to ≃ 20 mg IT. A total of 21 episodes were treated. In all but one case, neurological improvements both objectively and subjectively was obtained yielding approximately a 95% response rate.

Of the 14 evaluable patients, 7 had AML. Of these 7, 6 responded to IT methotrexate. Two of the cases were quite interesting and perhaps should be considered separately. Both Oldstone et al[46] and Kwaan et al[45] reported cases of CGL where one of the manifestations of metamorphosis to a

blastic phase of CGL was meningeal leukemia. In both cases
the patients responded to IT methotrexate.

It is interesting that for both ALL and AML the overall response rate in the treatment of meningeal leukemia
is ≃ 2-4 times that of systemic methotrexate when it is
used alone to treat peripheral leukemia. Perhaps one reason for this is that ≃ 10 times higher concentration of the
antifolic agent can be attained in the CSF without causing
systemic toxitity. If one attempted to achieve the levels
in the serum that are present in the CSF after a single
instillation of methotrexate IT, one would almost certainly encounter lethal toxicity.

REFERENCES

1. Farber, S., et al. Temporary remission in acute leukemia
   in children produced by folic acid antagonist,
   4-aminopteroyl-glutamic acid (Aminopterin). New Eng J
   Med 238: 787, 1948.

2. Sansone, G. Pathomorphosis of acute infantile leukemia
   treated with modern therapeutic agents; "Meningoleukemia" and "Frolich's Obesity". Ann Pediat (Basel)
   183: 33, 1954.

3. Bertino, J. The mechanism of action of the folate
   antagonists in man. Cancer Res 23: 1286, 1963.

4. Werkheiser, W. The biochemical, cellular, and pharmacological action and effects of the folic acid antagonists. Cancer Res 23: 1277, 1963.

5. Roberts, D., and Wodinsky, I. On the poor correlation
   between the inhibition by methotrexate of dihydrofolate
   reductase and of deoxynucleoside incorporation into
   RNA. Cancer Res 28: 1955, 1968.

6. Fischer, G. Increased levels of folic acid reductase
   as a mechanism of resistance to amethopterin in leukemic cells. Biochem Pharmacol 7: 75, 1961.

7. Hakala, M., Lakrzewski, S., and Nichol, C. Relation
   of folic acid reductase to amethopterin resistance
   in cultured mammalian cells. J Biol Chem 236: 952,
   1961.

8. Hakala, M. On the role of drug penetration in amethopterin resistance of Sarcoma-180 cells in vitro Biochem Biophys Acta 102: 198, 1965.

9. Kessel, D., and Hall, T., Roberts, D., et al. Modification of treatment schedules in the management of ad
   vanced mouse leukemia with amethopterin. J Nat Cancer
   Inst 17: 203, 1956.

10. Welch, A.D. The problem of drug resistance in cancer chemotherapy. Cancer Res 19: 359,, 1959.

11. Nichol, C.A. Studies of the mechanism of resistance to folic acid antagonists by leukemic cells. Cancer Res 14: 522, 1954.

12. Nichol, C.A. Studies on resistance to folic acid antagonists. In J.W. Rebuck, F.H. Bethell, and R.W. Monto. The leukemias: Etiology, pathophysiology and treatment. New York, Academic Press, Inc., 583, 1957.

13. Nichol, C.A., Welch, A.D. Metabolic requirements for formation of citrovorum factor and studies of mechanism of resistance to amethopterin. In Antimetabolites and Cancer. An Assn Adv Science, New York, 1965.

14. Law, L. W. Differences between cancers in terms of evolution of drug resistance. Cancer Res 16: 698, 1956.

15. Whiteside, J.A., Philips, F.S., Dargeon, H.W., and Burchenal, J.H. Intrathecal amethopterin in neurological manifestations of leukemia. Arch Intern Med 101: 279, 1958.

16. Hyman, C.B., Brubaker, C.A., and Sturgeon, P. Intrathecal methotrexate in the treatment of CNS complications of acute leukemia. W Soc Clin Res 7: 93, 1959.

17. Cramblett, H.G. Recognition and treatment of intracranial manifestations of leukemia. Amer J Dis Child 97: 805, 1959.

18. Murphy, M.L. Leukemia and lymphoma in children. Pediat Clin N Amer 6: 611, 1959.

19. Shaw, R.K., Moore, E.W., Freireich, E.J., and Thomas, L.B. Meningeal leukemia. A syndrome resulting from increased intracranial pressure in patients with acute leukemia. Neurology 10: 823, 1960.

20. Laurance, B.M. Intracranial complications of leukaemia treated with intrathecal amethopterin. Arch Dis Child 36: 107, 1961.

21. Zimmerman, V.H., Zum problem der meningealen leukamie und der meningealen reticulose. Schweiz Med Wsch 91: 1555, 1961.

22. Cottom, D.G., and Wetherley-Mein, G. Leukaemic meningitis. Arch Dis Child 36: 424, 1961.

23. Pierce, M.I. Neurologic complications in acute leukemia in children. Pediat Clin N Amer 9: 425, 1962.

24. Steffey, J.M. The central nervous system manifestations
    of leukemia. A report of 6 cases with meningeal in-
    volvement. J Pediat 60: 183, 1962.

25. Wegelius, R., Michelsson, K., and Wasz-Hockert, O.
    Acute leukemia in children. A review of 229 cases
    treated according to different principles. Ann
    Paediat Fenn 9: 86, 1963.

26. Evans, A.E. Central nervous system involvement in
    children with acute leukemia. Cancer 17: 256, 1963.

27. Haghbin, M., and Zuelzer, W.W. A long-term study of
    cerebrospinal leukemia. J Pediat 67: 23, 1965.

28. Yakar, D., and Padeh, B. Acute leukemia with meningeal
    involvement. Proc Tel-Hashomer Hosp (Tel-Aviv) 5: 63
    1966.

29. Koch, K., Reiquam, C.W., and Beatty, E.C., Jr. Acute
    childhood leukemia. Unusual complications. Rocky
    Mountain Med J 63: 50, 1966.

30. Hardisty, R.M., and Norman, P.M. Meningeal leukaemia.
    Arch Dis Child 42: 411, 1967.

31. Peter, A., Romhanyi, J., and Letenyei, K. Cerebro-
    spinal fluid diagnosis of meningeal leukaemia. Haema-
    tologia (Budapest) 1: 181, 1967.

32. Falkson, G., Van Eden, E.B., and Falkson, H.C. Menin-
    geal leukaemia. Med Proc (Johannesburg) 15: 13, 1968.

33. Selawry, O.S., and Odom, S. On eradication of leukemic
    meningopathy. Proc Amer Assoc Cancer Res 9: 62, 1968.

34. Sullivan, M.P., Vietti, T.J., Fernbach, D.J., Griffith,
    K.M., Haddy, T.B., and Watkins, W.L. Clinical inves-
    tigations in the treatment of meningeal leukemia:
    radiation therapy regimens vs conventional intrathecal
    methotrexate. Blood 34: 301, 1969.

35. Sullivan, M.P., Haggard, M.E., Donaldson, M.H., and
    Krall, J. Comparison of the prolongation of remission
    in meningeal leukemia with maintenance intrathecal
    methotrexate (IT MTX) and intravenous bis-nitrosourea
    (BCNU). Proc Amer Assn Cancer Res 11: 77, 1970.

36. Kanner, S.P., Wiernik, P.H., Serpick, A.A., and
    Walker, M.D. CNS leukemia mimicking multifocal
    leukoencephalopathy. Amer J Dis Child 119: 264, 1970.

37. Nies, B.A., Thomas, L.B., and Freireich, E.J. Men-
    ingeal leukemia, a follow-up study. Cancer 18(5):
    546, 1965.

38. Shanbrom, E., Miller, S., and Fairbanks, V.F. Intrathecal administration of amethopterin in leukemic encephalopathy of young adults. New Eng J Med 265: 169, 1961.

39. Baker, G.P., and Oliver, R.A.M. Neurological complications of acute leukaemia in remission. Lancet 1: 837, 1962.

40. Soscia, J.L., Di Benedetto, R., Crocco, J., and Komninos, Z.D. Treatment of "leukemic encephalopathy" with intrathecal amethopterin. Dis Nerv Syst 25: 308, 1964.

41. Spiers, A.S.D., and Clubb, J.S. Meningeal involvement in acute leukaemia of adults, with a report on a patient treated by methotrexate intrathecally administered. Med J Aust 1: 930, 1966.

42. MacDougall, R.W.A. Neurological complications of acute leukemia in an adult. J Neurol Sci 1: 291, 1964.

43. Baikie, A.G., and Spiers, A.S.D. Methotrexate in meningeal leukaemia. Lancet 2: 259, 1967.

44. Suh, K.S., and Shanks, J.R. Methotrexate in meningeal leukaemia. Lancet 2: 1042, 1967.

45. Kwaan, H.C., Pierre, R.V., and Long, D.L. Meningeal involvement as first manifestation of acute myeloblastic transformation in chronic granulocytic leukemia. Blood 33: 348, 1969.

46. Oldstone, M.B.A., Wisotzkey, H., and Lau, T. Effect of intrathecally administered methotrexate on the central nervous system of man: report of three cases. Univ Md Sch Med Bull 53: 9, 1968.

B. Folic Acid Antagonists

2. Intrathecal Aminopterin

TABLE I
Intrathecal Aminopterin in Meningeal Leukemia

Reference	# pts.	Leukemia type ALL	Leukemia type AML	Sex M F	# episodes	Age yrs.	Hematol. CR	Hematol. PR	Status Rel.
Sansone, G., 1954[1]	2	2		2	2	9,12	1		1
Rieselbach, R.E., 1963[2]	15	15		7 8	24	4 yrs. mean	8		7
Nies, B.A. et al, 1965[3]	27				31	chil- dren	11	3	24

Intrathecal aminopterin was used intrathecally in a considerably fewer number of patients (See Table I). Sansone[1] was the first to use it in 1954. Rieselbach[2] noted that the drug has 5-10 times the antifolic activity of methotrexate and no significant increase in neurotoxicity when given intrathecally in dogs. He administered the drug to 15 patients in 24 different episodes of meningeal leukemia. The dosage was $\simeq 2.4$ mg/m^2 in divided doses. All the patients treated with this regimen had complete amelioration of symptoms and a return of the CSF to normal values. The remissions so induced lasted a median of about two months. Two of the patients had a complete bone marrow remission after 6 weeks of treatment with only IT aminopterin.

Nies[3] treated 31 episodes of meningeal leukemia with a dose of $\simeq 2.5$ mg/m^2 every week. The majority of his patients were in relapse. Objective CSF remissions were induced in 29 patients and all the patients treated had amelioration of symptoms and signs. The median duration of remission was $\simeq 9$ weeks.

Thus we have three studies which describe the use of aminopterin in $\simeq 44$ patients. The results of treatment are summarized in Table II. It would appear that in this smaller group of patients the drug is at least as effective as methotrexate in the treatment of meningeal leukemia. Whether the response rate is significantly different from methotrexate would be difficult to determine without comparative prospective studies.

TABLE I

Intrathecal Aminopterin in Meningeal Leukemia

IT Dose	Objective Response CR	PR	NC	Subjective Response CR	PR	NC	Duration of CNS Remission after Rx.	Duration of Leukemia after Rx.	Survival
0.036 mg/kg x 6 0.025 mg/kg x 2	2			1	1				12,16 mos.
2.4 mg/m² divided 24 doses	24			24			med. 2 mos.		
2.5 mg/m² QW	28	1	2	31			med 2 1/4 mos.		

TABLE II

Intrathecal Aminopterin

	# Pts.	# Episodes	Objective CR	PR	NC	Subjective CR	PR	NC
Evaluated by both Objective CSF remission and Subjective remission in signs and symptoms	44	57	52	3	2	55	1	1
% of Episodes			91%	5%	4%	98%	1%	1%
Overall response rate			96%			99%		
Combined response rate				97.5%				

REFERENCES

1. Sansone, G. Pathomorphosis of acute infantile leuke-
    mia treated with modern therapeutic agents; "Menin-
    goleukemia" and "Frolich's Obesity". Ann Pediat
    (Basel) 183: 33, 1954.

2. Rieselbach, R.E., et al. Intrathecal aminopterin
    therapy of meningeal leukemia. Arch Int Med 3:
    620, 1963.

3. Nies, B.A., Thomas, L.B., and Freireich, E.J. Menin-
    geal leukemia, a follow-up study. Cancer 18(5): 546,
    1965.

B. Folic Acid Antagonists

3. Intrathecal Antifolate Toxicity

The use of IT methotrexate or other antifolic agent,
is not without toxicity either local or systemic. Generally,
toxicity seen with IT methotrexate can be separated broad-
ly into two types. One is the morbidity one may encounter
by use of the procedure itself such as infection or bleeding.
The other is referable to the toxic effects of the drug
either locally or distant. The toxic effects of the drug
can be further subdivided into either idiosyncratic or dose
related.

It is well known that when antifolics are used to the
limits of toxicity one may see stomatitis, diarrhea, skin
and mucous membrane hemorrhage, pancytopenia, and alopecia[1].
The induced folate deficiency may lead to megaloblastic
anemia. Whiteside et al[2], in dogs, found that IT methotrexate
could be tolerated up to 0.5 mg/kg. At this dose there was
a megaloblastosis and a mild depression of the total
nucleated cell count in the marrow. A dose of 1.8 mg/kg
in one dog was lethal, presumably due to prolonged serum
levels which produced systemic toxicity similar to that
seen after oral administrations of frequent large doses
of methotrexate. It would appear that amethopterin from
the spinal depot is released slowly into the blood to give
these prolonged levels.

Sansone[3] used IT aminopterin at a dose of 0.025 mg x 2
days in one patient and 0.036 mg x 6 days in another patient
without obvious systemic effects. Whiteside[2], based on the
aforementioned experiments in dogs, used 0.5 mg/kg in
children with meningeal leukemia, and found it to be well
tolerated. Megaloblastosis was noted 7-10 days after instillation of methotrexate. In two of the patients, the bone
marrow revealed over 50% megaloblasts. No other side effects
were mentioned. Cramblett[4] in that same year noted no unusual immediate undesirable side effects of IT methotrexate
therapy. Murphy[5] gave up to 10 injections of 0.5 mg/kg IT
without harm.

Since that time, as evidenced by the plethora of papers
describing its use, IT methotrexate has been used in hun-
dreds of patients without a significantly high incidence
of side effects. The amount of methotrexate given IT is
quantitatively about the same dose which is given systemically. One would, therefore, expect the appearance of systemic toxicity, especially if the patients had also been
receiving methotrexate by mouth. Indeed, with higher CSF
levels of antifolic activity, systemic toxicity would be
a dose limiting factor. However, Wollner et al[6] demonstrated

in dogs that systemic toxicity from IT administered folic
acid antagonists may be avoided by concurrent intramuscular
injections of citrovorum factor, (leucovrin) which is essen-
tially excluded from cerebrospinal fluid. Although leucovorin does not displace methotrexate from the reductase,
it provides a utilizable form of THF that cells can con-
vert into the various essential coenzyme forms. Since
leucovorin does not penetrate into the CSF, one could use
larger doses IT and rescue the periphery. Pierce[7], described two children who had been under treatment with methotrexate orally until the meningeal signs were detected. On
the second day following IT methotrexate buccal lesions,
leukopenia, and skin rash appeared. The signs of toxicity
were controlled by the prompt administration of leucovorin,
3 mg intramuscularly, at intervals of 12 hours for three
injections.

Rieselbach[8] used the principle of leucovorin rescue in
the treatment of seven episodes in five patients with
doses of aminopterin exceeding systemic tolerance. These
ranged from 3.5-15.0 mg/m^2; the median of 23 treatments
was 12 mg/m^2. Potentially lethal systemic toxicity was
averted by concurrent intramuscular citrovorum factor
administration in a dose 10 times that of aminopterin. No
gastrointestinal toxicity or hematological effect was
noted at any time, as compared with an incidence of 64%
GI toxicity in patients receiving 3 mg/m^2 IT aminopterin
without leucovorin. It is interesting that as much as 52
mg of methotrexate has been given intrathecally (inadvert-
ently) without neurotoxicity. In that case, leucovorin
rescue was used and no signs of systemic toxicity appeared.

Hyman[9], in 1965, noted that systemic toxicity occurred
during six of sixty-seven courses of IT methotrexate. In
no instance was the toxicity fatal although in two hema-
topoietic toxicity depression was severe and required
supportive therapy.

Sullivan[10], in 1966, described the side effects of
IT methotrexate which occurred in 36 children receiving
54 courses of therapy. The drug treatment employed con-

TABLE I
Side Effects of IT MTX[10]

# Pts.	# Episodes	Fever	Mouth Ulcers	Rash	Meningeal Signs [a]	Head aches	Vomiting	CSF Pres. [b]	Conv. sions	Jaund- ice
36	54	11	11	6	10	10	15	11	2	2
% of Episodes		20%	20%	11%	19%	19%	28%	20%	4%	4%

a↑ denotes increase
b↓ denotes decrease

sisted of methotrexate 0.5 mg/kg of body weight (not to
exceed 15 mg per treatment) every other day until the
spinal fluid white cell count fell to below 10 cells/mm^3.
The total doses ranged from 0.28 mg/kg up to 8.0 mg/kg.
Table I is a summary of the types of toxicity found.

Anorexia and listlessness, unassociated with other
symptoms, were noted in one treatment case. One of the
54 courses of therapy of IT methotrexate resulted in
megaloblastosis; leukopenia was seen in two courses;
systemic antileukemic effect in three courses. In 26 of
54 (48%) courses of therapy, the combination of increasing meningeal signs, increasing headaches, and increase
in vomiting were interpreted as symptoms suggestive of
chemical arachnoiditis. Rising spinal fluid protein
levels were noted in 75% of the courses in which two or
more IT treatments were given. One patient experienced
pain in the legs and subsequently developed paraplegia.

In addition to the toxicity described heretofore,
idiosyncratic reactions resulting in death have been reported in the literature. The first such case was reported in 1969 by Back[11]. The patient was an 11 year old girl
who had previously completed two courses of IT methotrexate
therapy and was undergoing her final dose on the third
course of therapy. Approximately half of the methotrexate
had been injected when she complained of severe pain in her
left leg and abdomen. The injection was discontinued. She
subsequently developed an urticarial rash, a sensory level
below the nipples, and no muscle power in the legs. About
1/2 hour later she had a cardiac arrest. Necropsy showed
no anatomical cause of death and the authors concluded
that the patient had an acute hypersensitivity reaction to
methotrexate.

Bagshawe et al[12] described three cases of transient
pain, anesthesia, or paresis in three cases that received
IT methotrexate. Most of the effects, however, were transi-
tory in nature lasting at the most two days.

Other possibilities for toxicity include those effects
which could be caused by the lumbar puncture alone.
Rieselbach[8] mentioned in his paper that although patients
were frequently thrombopenic or severely neutropenic, the
only complication which occurred after over 250 lumbar
punctures was one case of bacterial meningitis. Shaw et al[13]
performed 15 lumbar punctures on patients whose platelet
counts were below 10,000 per cubic millimeter but no bleeding problems developed. Bagshawe et al[12] described a common difficulty in patients who have had multiple lumbar
punctures, failure of the spinal fluid to flow from the
needle. However, none of the patients had high spinal
fluid protein concentrations. Sullivan[10] mentioned that
rising protein levels were noted in 75% of the courses

of methotrexate in which two or more IT treatments were given. Perhaps toxicologic studies would show a chemically induced arachnoiditis if the appropriate chronic toxicological studies were done.

REFERENCES

1. Wintrobe, M.M. Clinical hematology. Philadelphia, Lea and Febiger, 1967.

2. Whiteside, J.A. Philips, F.S., Dargeon, H.W., and Burchenal, J.H. Intrathecal amethopterin in neurological manifestations of leukemia. Arch Int Med 101: 279, 1958.

3. Sansone, G. Pathomorphosis of acute infantile leukemia treated with modern therapeutic agents; "Meningoleukemia" and "Frolich's Obesity". Ann Pediat (Basel) 183: 33, 1954.

4. Cramblett, H.G. Recognition and treatment of intracranial manifestations of leukemia. Amer J Dis Child 97: 805, 1959.

5. Murphy, M.L. Leukemia and lymphoma in children. Pediat Clin N Amer 6: 611, 1959.

6. Wollner, N., Murphy, M.L., and Gordon, C.S. A study of intrathecal methotrexate, Abstract, Proc Amer Assn Cancer Res 3: 74, 1959.

7. Pierce, M.I. Neurologic complications in acute leukemia in children. Pediat Clin N Amer 9: 425, 1962.

8. Rieselbach, R.E., et al. Intrathecal aminopterin therapy of meningeal leukemia. Arch Int Med 3: 620, 1963.

9. Hyman, C.B., Bogle, J.M., Brubaker, C.A. Williams, K., and Hammond, D. Central nervous system involvement by leukemia in children. II. Therapy with intrathecal methotrexate. Blood 25: 13, 1965.

10. Sullivan, M.P., and Windmiller, J. Side effects of amethopterin (methotrexate) administered intrathecally in the treatment of meningeal leukemia. Med Rec Ann 59(3): 92, 1966.

11. Back, E.H. Death after intrathecal methotrexate. Lancet 2: 1005 , 1969.

12. Bagshawe, K.D., Magrath, I.T., and Golding, P.R. Intrathecal methotrexate. Lancet 2: 1258, 1969.

13. Shaw, R.K., Moore, E.W., Freireich, E.J., and Thomas,
     L.B. Meningeal leukemia. A syndrome resulting from
     increased intracranial pressure in patients with
     acute leukemia. Neurology 10: 823, 1960.

C. Ommaya-Pump Reservoir

As we have seen up to now, the therapy of meningeal leukemia has been limited to a great extent by barriers. Significantly, the functional anatomy of the cranial vault causes symptoms and signs of increased intracranial pressure which are difficult to ameliorate surgically. The unique physiology and microscopic anatomy implied in the concept of the "blood-brain barrier", limits the entry of many chemotherapeutic agents from blood to brain and, by doing so, makes systemic chemotherapy inadequate.

The most promising method to date has been the IT application of drugs via lumbar puncture. Most recently, however, a system was devised utilizing CSF pathways for the continuous and restricted delivery of high concentrations of chemotherapeutic agents from ventricular and spinal fluid to brain; the Ommaya-pump apparatus.

The technique utilizes a silicon rubber cannula with an attached reservoir, and is inserted surgically into the frontal horn of a lateral ventricle. Through this cannula one may then either inject or perfuse chemotherapeutic agents at will without having to resort to repeated lumbar punctures. This method was first described by Ommaya et al in 1963[1].

In 1965, Rubin et al[2], described the use of the Ommaya-pump reservoir in the perfusion of the CSF in children with meningeal leukemia. The experiment involves placing the cannula into the frontal horn of a lateral ventricle, perfusing the ventricular system with 10 to $\simeq$ 40 γ/ml of drug at a rate of $\simeq$ 1.5-1.9 ml/min and collecting

TABLE I
Complications of Reservoir Use[3]

Complications	# of Patients
Failure to function	14
Positive culture of cerebrospinal fluid from reservoirs without clinical infection	5
Seizures - well controlled with medication	3
Seizures - uncontrolled	2
Bacterial meningitis	4
Aseptic meningitis	2
Cellulitis without removal of reservoir	1

TABLE II
Ommaya-Pump Reservoir

Reference	# Pts.	Leukemia Type ALL	AML	Sex M	F	# episodes	yrs. age	Hematol. Status CR	PR	Rel.
Rubin et al, 1965[2]	2	2				2	children	2		
Ratcheson et al, 1966[3]	3					3	children			

the perfusate via a permanent lumbar cannula and reservoir. Their series includes two patients with meningeal leukemia who were symptomatic with headache and demonstrated a pleocytosis in the spinal fluid. Both were in systemic remission and had failed to respond to repeated IT aminopterin. Both patients experienced symptomatic relief and disappearance of their pleocytosis. At the time of the publication, one patient was still alive and one patient died of an unrelated cause. At postmortem, in that patient, no identifiable leukemic cells were found within the central nervous system. A granular ependymitis was evident, however, in many areas of the ventricular system.

In 1968, Ratcheson and Ommaya[3] reported on the use of the Ommaya-pump in 60 patients with various intracranial neoplasms. They included three patients with meningeal leukemia perfused with aminopterin. Of these three patients, two had a beneficial effect while in one a detrimental effect was seen due to complications with the technique. In Table I is shown the complications of reservoir use in 60 patients.

It becomes readily apparent that the use of the reservoir is often fraught with serious complications. Of significance especially is the high rate of bacterial meningitis ($\simeq$ 8%). This is very much higher than that seen with LP alone in meningeal leukemia (only one reported case in the literature) and is a potentially lethal complication if it occurs in this group of patients.

Based on the reported experience to date in Table II, there is an approximately 80% response. This technique appears to offer little to recommend it over standard IT therapy. Improvements in this system with added experience and refinement may yet show it to have a significant place in therapy, however.

TABLE II

Ommaya-Pump Reservoir

IT Dose	Objective Response CR PR NC			Subjective Response CR PR NC			Duration of CNS Remission after Rx.	Duration of Leukemia after Rx.	Survival
MTX 10-40 mcg/ml 1.5-1.9 ml/min	2			2					
Aminopterin	2		1	2		1			

REFERENCES

1. Ommaya, A.K. Subcutaneous reservoir and pump for sterile access to ventricular cerebrospinal fluid. Lancet 2: 983, 1963.

2. Rubin, R.C., Ommaya, A.K., Henderson, E.S., Bering, E.A., and Rall, D.P. Cerebrospinal fluid perfusion for central nervous system neoplasms. Neurology 16: 680, 1966.

3. Ratcheson, R.A., and Ommaya, A.K. Experience with subcutaneous cerebrospinal-fluid reservoir. Preliminary report of 60 cases. New Eng J Med 279: 1025, 1968.

D. Cytosine Arabinoside

1-β-D-Arabinosuranosylcytosine (Ara-C) has been intensively developed over the last 10 years and is now generally accepted as a useful drug in the treatment of AML in adults. The drug specifically inhibits DNA polymerase[1] and has been shown to be S-phase specific. The drug shows schedule dependency in the L1210 tumor system and is most active (ILS of 400%) when given every three hours on a day 1, 5, 9 schedule.

Cytosine arabinoside was early recognized in mice to pass the blood-brain barrier and to affect leukemia which was inoculated intracerebrally. In the clinical situation, substantial evidence of this has not been seen, although the drug has not been studied vigorously in this regard.

Owens, from the Roswell Park Group, was one of the first to administer Ara-C into dogs intrathecally[2]. He found that IT Ara-C did not produce toxic effects in dogs up to 11 doses. Walker and Rall[2] studied Ara-C by IT perfusion in dogs and monkeys and found that doses up to 22 mg/m^2 in the dog, and 24 mg/m^2 in the monkey, produced no toxic effects. However, when the dose was doubled to 48 mg/m^2 two of three dogs died, not from abnormalities in the nervous system that were recognized, nor hematological factors, but from some wasting metabolic disease with anorexia. To date this type of toxicity has not been seen clinically.

TABLE I
IT Cytosine Arabinoside in Meningeal Leukemia

Reference	# Pts.	Leukemia Type ALL	AML	Sex M	F	# episodes	yrs. age	Hematol. Status CR	PR	Rel.
Holland et al, 1969[2]	17					17	child			
Wang et al, 1970[3]	13	11	2			15	child.	8		5
Halkowski, B. et al, 1970[4]	4					6	child.			

To date, Dr. Holland and Acute Leukemia Group B have treated 19 patients[2]. Seventeen of these 19 were evaluable and received between 5-50 mg/m^2 total dose IT. There were 6 complete responses lasting a median of $\simeq$ 2.5 plus months, very similar to the duration of remission seen for IT methotrexate. There were also four partial responses in the group. A very definite dose-response curve resulted with most of the responses seen at the higher dose levels. Indeed, Dr. Holland recommended a dose in the range of 20-30 mg/m^2. There was no thrombocytopenia or leukopenia that could be attributed to the drug, for rapid deamination occurs on exiting from the CSF. In summary, they believed that Ara-C offers an alternative treatment for patients with CNS leukemia with definite therapeutic usefulness.

In early 1971, two more reports have appeared describing the IT use of Ara-C. Wang and Pratt[3] treated 13 patients with Ara-C IT, 11 with ALL and two with AML. Eight of the patients with ALL were in remission while the remaining patients with ALL and the two patients with AML were in hematological relapse. The drug drug was diluted with Elliot's B solution and administered in dosages ranging from 5 to 70 mg/m^2. Of the 11 patients with ALL, seven responded both objectively and subjectively. Five of these patients were in hematological remission while two were in hematological relapse. The median duration of response was about one month. The two patients with AML showed no response to the drug. This is surprising in light of the recent reports of favorable effects of Ara-C in systemic AML. Toxicity included nausea, vomiting, headache, and fever. No child experienced serious neurologic complications or myelo-suppression. It is interesting that seven of the children with ALL had previously been treated with cranial or craniospinal irradiation while two of the patients with ALL had prednisone resistant meningeal leukemia. Four of

TABLE I
IT Cytosine Arabinoside in Meningeal Leukemia

IT Dose	Objective Response CR	PR	NC	Subjective Response CR	PR	NC	Duration of CNS Remission after Rx.	Duration of Leukemia after Rx.	Survival
5-50 mg/m^2	6	4	7	6	4	7	med. 2.5 mos.		
5-70 mg/m^2	8		7	8		7	med. 1.0 mos.		
IT MTX 0.1-1.6 mg/kg x 2-4 IT Ara-C 0.8-2.2 mg/kg x 2-4	6			6					

the seven patients who had previously been treated with irradiation responded to therapy.

Halkowski et al[4], in 1970, reported on the combination of IT methotrexate and IT Ara-C. The methotrexate dose was 0.1-1.6 mg/kg x 2-4 doses and Ara-C dose was 0.8-2.2 mg/kg x 2-4 doses. Both were administered concurrently. Four patients were treated who had a total of 6 episodes. All 6 episodes responded to this regimen. That the treatment was effective is interesting on theoretical grounds, since methotrexate would tend to be self-limiting and hold cells in G1 and G2. This would restrict the cells from entering S where Ara-C exhibits its effect.

In summary then, (Table I), of 30 patients (32 episodes) treated with only Ara-C, there were 18 responses yielding a response rate of $\simeq$ 56%. With the combination of Ara-C and methotrexate, 10 patients (12 episodes) have been treated with 11 responses for an overall response rate of better than 90%. These results are comparable with both IT methotrexate and radiotherapy, but not superior to these modes of therapy. What is perhaps more significant is that Ara-C may be used in those cases that prove refractory to the more conventional modes of therapy.

REFERENCES

1. Furth, J., and Cohen, S. Inhibition of mammalian DNA polymerase by the 5'-triphosphate of 1-β-D-arabinofuranosylcytosine and the 5'-triphosphate of 9-β-D-arabinofuranosyladenine. Cancer Res 28: 2061, 1968.

2. Holland, J. Use in childhood acute leukemia: central nervous system leukemia in children. In "Proceedings of the Chemotherapy Conference on Ara-C. Development and Application." (Carter, S.K., and Livingston, R.B., eds.), 1969.

3. Wang, J.J., and Pratt, C.B. Intrathecal arabinosyl cytosine in meningeal leukemia. Cancer 25: 531, 1970.

4. Halkowski, B., Cyklis, R., Armata, J., Garwicsz S., Wyszkowski, J., and Garapich, M. Cytosine arabinoside administered intrathecally in cerebromeningeal leukemia. Acta Pediat Scand 59: 164, 1970.

E. L-Asparaginase

L-Asparaginase is an enzyme produced by E. coli which
exerts antitumor activity through catalyzing the hydrolysis
of asparagine, thereby probably inhibiting synthesis of
vital proteins in sensitive cells (those which are incap-
able of synthesizing sufficient L-asparaginase for their
own needs, and are dependent therefore on an exogenous
supply). It appears to be especially effective in the
treatment of acute leukemias, primarily ALL as compared to
AML, and is of special importance in that there appears
to be no cross-resistance of tumors between L-asparaginase
and other chemotherapeutic agents[1]. Remissions induced by
the drug are often dramatic and complete, but appear to be
fairly short-lived, probably related to the survival and
proliferation of malignant cells with sufficient asparagine
synthetase activity to overcome the effects of deprivation
of an exogenous supply of the amino acid[1]. The systemic
toxicity seen with L-asparaginase includes: hepatic, in
the form of altered liver function tests, hypoalbuminemia,
fatty metamorphosis; hypocholesterolemia CNS with depression or excitation; altered clotting factors; pancreatitis;
hyperosmolar coma; elevated blood ammonia levels; it is
remarkably free of myelosuppression or GI tract toxicity[1].

Several tumors in mice, rats and dogs have been shown
to be sensitive to L-asparaginase[1]. However, mouse
L1210 leukemia is insensitive to the drug. It is interest-
ing that L-asparaginase will affect IC inoculated tumors.
Burchenal demonstrated, in mice bearing strain CA 55
leukemia inoculated IC, a 112-171% increase in survival.
These were in systemic doses ranging from 50-1,000 iu/kg
for 1-20 days. The total dose was always 1,000 iu/kg.
There was no schedule dependency exhibited for this tumor.
Perhaps breakdown of the "blood-brain barrier" by the
tumor allows the enzyme to enter the intracerebral and
CSF compartments.

In pharmacological studies done by Schwartz[2] in humans
without CNS leukemia, there was no detectable L-asparaginase in the CSF after systemic administration at a dose
of 200 iu/kg for up to 28 days. However, plasma levels
were directly related to the dose administered. Others,
using sensitive radioimmunoassay methods, have found that
the concentration of L-asparaginase in the CSF at equilib-
rium was 0.4 to 1% that of a simultaneous plasma level.
There is the possibility that even this small amount may
have an effect on meningeal leukemia, since often times
the cells are exquisitely sensitive to the effects of the
drug.

TABLE I
L-Asparaginase in the Treatment of Meningeal Leukemia

Reference	# Pts.	Leukemia Type		Sex		# episodes	yrs. age	Hematol. Status		
		ALL	AML	M	F			CR	PR	Rel.
Tallal et al, 1970[4]	13	13				13	chil-dren			13
	6					6	chil-dren			6
Tan et al, 1970[3]	7	7				7	5 children 2 adults			

Tan and Oettgen[3] recently reported that doses up to 5000 iu/kg IV did not produce detectable CSF levels in man. Clinical evidence however, suggests that the drug may enter the CSF in patients with CNS leukemia. Tallal et al[4], in 1971, reported on thirteen children who had evidence of CNS leukemia at the onset of enzyme treatment as manifested by pleocytosis and/or increased protein levels in the CSF, with or without clinical symptomatology. During the time the enzyme was being administered by daily IV or thrice weekly IM injections, significant objective improvement in the CNS was seen in six of the thirteen patients whose doses ranged from 10 to 1,000 iu/kg. Each of the six patients developed a bone marrow remission while none of the seven nonresponders achieved a bonemarrow remission.

In Tallal's[4] study, preliminary laboratory studies had shown the enzyme could be given intrathecally to dogs without causing significant toxic effects. Six additional patients were then given the drug IT in total doses ranging from 250 to 3,600 iu/kg over a period of 7 to 22 days. The enzyme was well tolerated causing no untoward reactions other than a transient inflammatory response (increased polymorphonuclear leukocytes and increased protein in the spinal fluid). Three out of the six patients responded with two complete responses and one partial response. The number of leukemic cells in the CSF was reduced only when they were also responsive in the bone marrow.

Tan and Oettgen[3] treated seven more patients with IT L-asparaginase in doses of 100-5,000 iu daily. All the patients had ALL and there were five children and two adults in the group. After intraventricular administration the enzyme was found promptly in the CSF obtained by LP and also appeared in the plasma. Thus it appears at least that the enzyme can go from CSF to plasma. It is also becoming clearer why the drug was not found in the CSF in the study done by Schwartz[2]; none of the patients had meningeal leukemia. Of the five children treated with the

TABLE I

L-Asparaginase in the Treatment of Meningeal Leukemia

Dose	Objective Response			Subjective Response			Duration of CNS Remission after Rx.	Duration of Leukemia after Rx.	Survival
	CR	PR	NC	CR	PR	NC			
10-1,000 IU/kg IV	6		7						
250-3,600 IU/kg IT	2	1	3						
1,000-5,000 IU QD IT	3		1				transient		

drug IT, three showed transient improvement in CSF parameters, one was given interval treatment and could not be
evaluated, and one did not respond. The two adults treated
could not be evaluated since their treatments were started
recently. In all of the patients the treatment was well
tolerated.

In summary then, 26 patients have been treated with
L-asparaginase either IV or IT (Table I). In both cases the
overall response rate is ≃ 50%. Significantly, in the IV
administered cases, if there was not a concomitant bone
marrow response, there was no CSF response. The use of
L-asparaginase, since it shows no therapeutic advantage
over the other conventional modes of therapy probably
should be limited only to those patients who are refractory to other therapy.

REFERENCES

1. Livingston, R.B., and Carter, S.K. L-Asparaginase Clinical
    brochure. Cancer Therapy Evaluation Branch, NCI, 1969.

2. Schwartz, M.K., Lash, E.D., Oettgen, H.F., and Tomao,
    F.A. L-asparaginase activity in plasma and other bio-
    logical fluids. Cancer 25: 244, 1970.

3. Tan, C., and Oettgen, H. Clinical experience with
    L-asparaginase administered intrathecally. Proc Amer
    Assoc Cancer Res 10: 92, 1969.

4. Tallal, L., Tan, C., Oettgen, H., Wollner, N., McCarthy,
    M., Helson, L., Burchenal, J., Karnofsky, D., and
    Murphy, M.L. E. coli L-asparaginase in the treatment
    of leukemia and solid tumors in 131 children. Cancer
    25: 306, 1970.

F. Corticosteroids

TABLE I
IT Steroids in the Treatment of Meningeal Leukemia

Reference	# Pts.	Leukemia Type ALL	AML	Sex M	F	# episodes	yrs. age	Hematol. CR	Status PR	Rel.
Dost, 1956[2]	1					1	child			

The use of IT corticosteroids in man has had a long history, primarily in the treatment of non-malignant disease. This mode of administration of steroids has been advocated as therapy for adhesive arachnoiditis, tuberculous meningitis, multiple sclerosis and other neurological disorders[1]. In these reports, the water insoluble derivatives of cortisone and hydrocortisone have been used with dosages being quite low, 1-2 mg/kg or less.

Since parenteral administration or withdrawal of these agents may be associated with convulsions, and since these drugs do have definite effects on the excitability of the central nervous system Oppelt and Rall[1] decided to study these drugs IT. They found that IT administration of soluble hydrocortisone succinate in doses of 2.25 to 6 mg/kg and soluble prednisolone-21-phosphate in doses of 1.5 mg/kg resulted in severe convulsions in dogs. Neither insoluble hydrocortisone suspension in saline, nor a sodium phosphate buffer similar to the one in which the hydrocortisone succinate is dissolved, had a deleterious effect. They cautioned about the use of these drugs in human beings.

There is only one reference to the use of IT adrenal steroids alone in the treatment of meningeal leukemia (see Table I). This was in 1956 by Dost[2], who found a response in a child with meningeal leukemia.

Since then, perhaps due to the hesitancy to use steroid IT or the availability of other agents in the treatment of meningeal leukemia, there has not been much interest in the drug intrathecally. However, just recently the Southwest Group has placed patients on a protocol involving the use of IT methotrexate plus IT hydrocortisone in doses of 10 mg/m^2 and 6 mg/m^2 respectively until the CSF WBC drops to <10 cells/mm^3. The results of this protocol are still preliminary.

TABLE I
IT Steroids in the Treatment of Meningeal Leukemia

IT Dose	Objective Response CR PR NC	Subjective Response CR PR NC	Duration of CNS Remission after Rx.	Duration of Leukemia after Rx.	Survival
	1	1			

REFERENCES

1. Oppelt, W.W., and Rall, D.P. Production of convulsions
    in the dog with intrathecal corticosteroids. Neurology
    11(10): 925, 1961.

2. Dost, F.H. Leukamische menigopathic und iridopathic
    beim. Kind Arzt Wochen 11: 1070, 1956.

V. RADIOTHERAPY

Irradiation as a treatment for meningeal leukemia has been used for many years. D'Angio[1] began to use radiotherapy as early as 1953. At one point during the late 50's, it was considered the treatment of choice for meningeal leukemia. Prior to 1953 there was a long historical experience concerning the treatment of brain tumors with irradiation.

The animal data is interesting in that it does not correlate with the clinical results. Using radiotherapy alone Johnson[2], in 1962, did a rather definitive study comparing CNS radiation with control mice and mice systemically treated with Cytoxan. The model in the mice was the intracranially implanted L1210 leukemia. It was found that radiation to the craniospinal axis when given in doses varying from 500 to 3000 rads per week did not significantly prolong the median survival time in the mice. Cytoxan, given in various doses systemically prolonged the median survival time to ≃ 14 days. No long-term survivals for either group of treated mice were seen. It is interesting that when both irradiation and chemotherapy were given concomitantly, there was a tremendous increase in survival time. This experiment will be described in some detail later.

Although the treatment of brain tumors in children had been described previously, Pierce[3], in 1954, was one of the first to describe irradiation in the treatment of the intracranial complications of leukemia. The patient was a boy eight years of age with stem cell leukemia who was treated for his systemic disease with ACTH and 6-MP. While in clinical remission, he developed a severe headache and meningeal signs. A lumbar tap revealed a cell count of $1250/mm^3$, all of which were blast forms. Severe papilledema developed. Following therapy with roentgen rays to the base of the skull, signs of increased intracranial pressure disappeared and the CSF leukocyte count fell to about 1/2 the pretreatment value. Pancytopenia developed soon after however and the patient expired.

In 1957, Sullivan[4] described 5 cases of meningeal leukemia that she treated with cranial radiotherapy. The doses used varied from a total tumor dose of 100 to 450 r given over several days. Six episodes were treated and there were two objective good responses and two symptomatic good responses. She concluded that radiotherapy was the most effective method of treatment of meningeal leukemia. She recommended a total tumor dose of 250-500 r to be given over ≃ 7-70 days.

D'Angio[1], in 1959, reported on the treatment of 62
episodes of meningeal leukemia with cranial radiotherapy
in doses ranging from 70 to 1390 r. Forty-seven of 62
episodes so treated responded symptomatically for about
a 76% response rate. The best results were obtained with
treatment early in the development of the complications
and before irreversible changes, such as permanent cranial
nerve palsies, occurred. Lumbar puncture alone, in the
same series yielded about a 44% response rate in relief
of symptoms. Following roentgen therapy, the average period
before recurrence was three months while that of lumbar
puncture plus radiotherapy was about four months. Radio-
resistance did not seem to develop in the patients. Indeed,
one child responded well to six courses of roentgen treatment over a period of one year. Epilation was noted in many
of the patients receiving skull irradiation. On the basis
of the data, the authors felt that the method of choice in
the treatment of meningeal leukemia was lumbar puncture,
followed by roentgen therapy if the symptoms persist or
recur within a few days.

During the decade beginning about 1960, many more papers
were reported in the literature. On Table I the results of
all the studies have been listed. From this larger table,
I have summarized the results on Table II.

As can be seen, in Table II the combined response rate
of 63% is lower than that seen for IT methotrexate alone
by ≃ 20%. It is also apparent that the results here reveal
that there is a dichotomy between the subjective (symptoms
and signs) response of 82% and the objective (CSF response)
of 44%. This data is somewhat skewed since Sullivan's data
makes up a rather large percentage of the total objective
response rate. Nevertheless, in the methotrexate IT data,
which also includes Sullivan's observations, this dichotomy
is not seen. It is therefore imperative that when one
evaluates the results in the treatment of meningeal leukemia,
one must in the future look at both objective as well as
subjective responses.

A closer look at Sullivan's data in Table I reveals
that for both 500 r or 1000 r given to the cranium only,
the objective response rates in the two groups respectively
are 14% and 8%, while the subjective response is 85% and
75% respectively. Thus it becomes apparent that radiotherapy to the cranium at these doses is quite effective
in relieving the patient's symptoms but does not appreciably alter the CSF. However, when the 1000 r dose is
given both to the cranium and the spine the objective
and subjective responses are 92% and 77% respectively.
This suggests that radiotherapy to both the skull and the
spinal cord must be given to achieve a significant objective response. Myelosuppression was the only side effect
of radiation therapy of medical significance and could be
accurately assessed only in children in bone marrow remis-

TABLE I
Radiotherapy in the Treatment of Meningeal Leukemia

Reference	# Pts.	Leukemia Type		Sex		episodes	yrs. age	Hematol. Staus		
		ALL	AML	M	F			CR	PR	Rel.
Pierce, 1954[5]	1	stem cell		1		1	8	1		
Sullivan, 1957[4]	5		1			6	children	1		4
D'Angio et al, 1959[1]	37	37		20	17	62	children			
Shaw et al, 1960[6]	7					7	children			
Pierce, M.I., 1962[3]	10					10	av.4	5	3	2
Evans, A. et al, 1963[7]	53					50	children			
Haghbin, M. et al, 1965[8]	61			39	22	42	children			
Koch et al, 1967[10]	28					18	children			
Hardisty et al, 1967[10] 1970[0]	29			14	15	4	children			
Sullivan et al, 1969	7					7	children			
	12					12	children			
	13					13	children			

TABLE II
Cranial or Craniospinal Radiotherapy

	# Pts.	# Episodes
Evaluated Objectively	0	0
Evaluated Subjectively	135	147
Evaluated by both criteria	38	39
% of Episodes		
Overall response rate		
Combined reponse rate		

TABLE I

Radiotherapy in the Treatment of Meningeal Leukemia

RT Dose	Objective Response			Subjective Response			Duration of CNS remission after Rx.	Duration of Leukemia after Rx.	Survival
	CR	PR	NC	CR	PR	NC			
?		1		1			short		
100-450 r TD cranium	2		4	2		4	?		
70-1390 r TD cranium				47			3-4 mos.		
600-1000 r TD cranium				3	1		1-3 mos.		
400-2,000 r TD cranium				7		3		med. 6 mos.	med. 15 mos
400 r TD cranium				49			mean 2.8 mos.		
200 r cranium					?		med. 3.0 mos.		
				16	1	1			
500 r TD cranium	1		6	4	2	1	2 mos.		
1000 r TD	1		11	9		3	1 month		
1000 r TD craniospinal	12		1	10		3	1.5 mos.		

TABLE II

Cranial or Craniospinal Radiotherapy

Objective			Subjective		
CR	PR	NC	CR	PR	NC
			122	2	23
16	1	22	26	2	11
41%	3%	56%	80%	2%	18%
44%			82%		
63%					

sion. No marrow depression occurred at the 500 rad level
while only one of seven had myelosuppression at the 1000
rad level to the cranium. However, when the 1000 rads
were given to the craniospinal axis, six of seven children developed leukopenia with WBC going as low as
1000/mm^3 in two patients. The median day of the nadir of
WBC depression was on the twelfth day. Four of the seven
children developed thrombocytopenia with counts ranging
from 26,000 to 88,000/mm^3 and a median day of nadir at
the fifteenth day. Marrow recovery was documented within
six weeks of completion of CNS therapy provided relapse
did not supervene.

REFERENCES

1. D'Angio, G.J., Evans, A.E., and Mitus, A. Roentgen
   therapy of certain complications of acute leukemia
   in childhood. Amer J Roentgen 82: 541, 1959.

2. Johnson, R.E. An experimental therapeutic approach to
   L1210 leukemia in mice: combined chemotherapy and
   central nervous system irradiation. J Nat Cancer Inst
   32(6): 1333, 1964.

3. Pierce, M.I. Neurologic complications in acute leukemia
   in children. Pediat Clin N Amer 9: 425, 1962.

4. Sullivan, M.P. Intracranial complications of leukemia
   in children. Pediatrics 20: 757, 1957.

5. Pierce, M. Leukemia in children: treatment of 22 cases
   with 6-mercaptopurine. Ann N Y Acad Sci 60: 415, 1954.

6. Shaw, R.K., Moore, E.W., Freireich, E.J., and Thomas,
   L.B. Meningeal leukemia. A syndrome resulting from
   increased intracranial pressure in patients with acute
   leukemia. Neurology 10: 823, 1960.

7. Evans, A.E. Central nervous system involvement in
   children with acute leukemia. Cancer 17: 256, 1963.

8. Haghbin, M., and Zuelzer, W.W. A long-term study of
   cerebrospinal leukemia. J Pediat 67: 23, 1965.

9. Koch, K., Reiquam, C.W., and Beatty, E.C., Jr. Acute
   childhood leukemia. Unusual complications. Rocky Mountain Med J 63: 50, 1966.

10. Hardisty, R.M., and Norman, P.M. Meningeal leukaemia.
    Arch Dis Child 42: 411, 1967.

11. Sullivan, M.P., Vietti, T.J., Fernbach, D.J., Griffith,
    K.M., Haddy, T.B., and Watkins, W.L. Clinical inves-
    tigations in the treatment of meningeal leukemia:
    radiation therapy regimens vs conventional intrathecal
    methotrexate. Blood 34: 301, 1969.

VI. COMBINATION RADIOTHERAPY AND CHEMOTHERAPY IN MENINGEAL LEUKEMIA

As was pointed out previously[1], craniospinal irradiation in the mouse, as treatment for intracranially implanted L1210 leukemia does not alter the course of the disease in terms of survival. In those same experiments however, Johnson[1] also used a combination of systemically administered Cytoxan and electron-beam irradiation to the entire cerebrospinal axis. The median survival for the controls as well as for the group only treated with craniospinal radiation was 10 days. The maximum median survival with drug therapy alone (Cytoxan) at the optimal dosage was only 14 days. However, the combined therapy of drug and radiation resulted in a highly significant prolongation of survival (more than 300%) compared with that of mice treated with either drug or irradiation alone. It also produced 70% apparent cures (60-day survivors). They concluded that the possibility exists for the complete irradication of all leukemic cells through this combined approach. Indeed, we shall see from the work described later that these results may have application in the treatment of meningeal leukemia in man.

Most of the studies utilizing combinations of chemotherapy and radiotherapy for meningeal leukemia have been involved in the prophylaxis of the disease rather than in the attempt at cure once CNS involvement has occurred. There has been however one study where the modalities of IT methotrexate either alone or in combination with radiotherapy was compared[2]. In that study, Sullivan[2] specifically randomized patients between various combinations of CNS therapy. Each treatment group consisted of a radiotherapy group and an IT methotrexate group (0.5 mg/kg x 2-3 day intervals until CSF cell count was below $10/mm^3$

TABLE I
Various Combinations of CNS Therapy[2]

Treatment	XRT Regimen		MTX Regimen	
	% CNS Rem.	Duration of Remission	% CNS Rem.	Duration of Remission
Skull 500	14%	2 months	57%	3 months
Skull 1000	8%	1 month	75%	3 months
Skull & Spine 1000	92%	1 and 3/4 months	85%	1 month
Combination	100%	3 months	84%	3 and 1/4 months

The combination group consisted of craniospinal irradiation of ≈ 1000 rads and IT methotrexate in the usual dose. Table I derived from that paper is used to summarize her results.

It is suggestive but not conclusive that the combination group not only had a greater percentage of CNS remissions (100%) but also one of the longest durations of CNS remissions (3 months). In any case combination therapy certainly is not any worse than the other modes of therapy and would appear superior to any of the other therapies described in the previous sections of this review.

REFERENCES

1. Johnson, R.E. An experimental therapeutic approach to L1210 leukemia in mice: combined chemotherapy and central nervous system irradiation. J Nat Cancer Inst 32(6): 1333, 1964.

2. Sullivan, M.P., Vietti, T.J., Fernbach, D.J., Griffith, K.M., Haddy, T.B., and Watkins, W.L. Clinical investigations in the treatment of meningeal leukemia: radiation therapy regimens vs conventional intrathecal methotrexate. Blood 34: 301, 1969.

VII. CENTRAL NERVOUS SYSTEM INVOLVEMENT
BY BURKITT'S LYMPHOMA

Some of the neurological parallels between the CSF in malignant pleocytosis in CSF in Burkitt's lymphoma and meningeal leukemia have been pointed out in the literature. For example, Janota[1], in an autopsy study, reported central nervous system involvement in 21 of 25 patients dying of Burkitt's lymphoma in an 18 month period. Indeed, as in meningeal leukemia, the incidence of involvement of the central nervous system has increased in recent years[2]. Again, this may be due to increased awareness or due to the application of chemotherapeutic agents which prolongs survival. However, that increased awareness plays a role is evidenced by the presence of lymphoma cells in the CSF in ≃ 25% of newly diagnosed cases found by Ziegler at the Lymphoma Treatment Center of Mulago Hospital, Kampala[2].

As with meningeal leukemia, tumor cells may be found infiltrating the choroid plexus and meninges. In the meningeal form of the disease, tumor cells fill the subarachnoid space and extend into the brain along the Virchow-Robin spaces[2]. Perivascular infiltration, as in meningeal leukemia, can also occur. Unlike meningeal leukemia, oftentimes the tumor will erode into the base of the skull causing direct extension of tumor into the brain.

Signs and symptoms of meningeal involvement by Burkitt's lymphoma are quite similar to that observed in meningeal leukemia. In 27 patients with meningeal involvement, the following symptoms were observed[3]:

Symptoms	# patients
Mental changes	11
Itching of skin	3
Vomiting	1
Meningismus	1
Convulsions	3
Cranial Nerve lesions	5
Paraplegia	9

More than 60% of patients with Burkitt's lymphoma studied in Kenya had lymphoma cells in the CSF at some time during the course of their disease[2]. When the CSF has been evaluated, the CSF protein has been elevated and the sugar content low.

As with meningeal leukemia certain drugs with low lipid solubility and a high degree of ionization such as

TABLE I
Intrathecal Methotrexate in Burkitt's Lymphoma

Reference	# Pts.	# Episodes	yrs. age	Hematol. Status CR	PR	Rel.	IT Dose
Ziegler and Bluming, 1970[4]	38	5					10 mg/wk x 4
		12					15 mg/wk x 4
		10					15 mg/wk x 10

TABLE II
Intrathecal Cytosine Arabinoside in Burkitt's Lymphoma

Reference	# Pts.	# Episodes	yrs. age	Hematol. Status CR	PR	Rel.	IT Dose
Ziegler and Bluming, 1970[4]	38	3					Ara-C 10-50 mg QW x 4
		15					MTX 25 mg alternating Ara-C 50 mg Q 4 days
		7					Ara-C 30 mg QD x 4
		5					Ara-C 30 mg QD x 10

methotrexate, Cytoxan, and others are of little value when the central nervous system is involved due to the inability of these agents to cross the blood-brain barrier. Clifford et al[3] utilized various agents systemically in an attempt to treat the CNS disease. These drugs included nitrogen mustard (HN_2), Cytoxan, Mannitol Myleran, methyl hydrazine, orthomerphalan, and chlorambucil. There was only one transient response to chlorambucil at a dose of 5 mg/kg/day x 1 day, possibly due to shrinkage of an extradural tumor. Thirteen additional patients were treated with BCNU or IT methotrexate or both of these drugs. Serial CSF determinations showed a falling of the tumor cell count in 4 patients, all of whom had received at least three injections of IT methotrexate.

Ziegler and Bluming[4] have recently treated a large number of patients with malignant pleocytosis secondary to Burkitt's lymphoma. This was encountered in ≈ 45% of their their patients with Burkitt's lymphoma in the past three years. They have treated 27 episodes of malignant pleocytosis in 38 patients with Burkitt's lymphoma utilizing

TABLE I

Intrathecal Methotrexate in Burkitt's Lymphoma

Objective Response CR PR NC	Subjective Response CR PR NC	Duration of CNS Remission after Rx.	Duration of Leukemia after Rx.	Survival
5	5			2 alive 3 yrs.
12	12	med. 5 mos.		
10	10	med. 3/4 month		

TABLE II

Intrathecal Cytosine Arabinoside in Burkitt's Lymphoma

Objective Response CR PR NC	Subjective Response CR PR NC	Duration of CNS Remission after Rx.	Duration of Leukemia after Rx.	Survival
3	3			
13	13			
7	7	med. 3.5 mos.		
5	5	med. 0.5 mos.		

three different methotrexate regimens as outlined in Table I. As can be seen, all of the regimens produced complete responses in this group of patients. However, in those patients receiving the high dose methotrexate regimen for 4 days, a clearly better response in terms of duration of remission was obtained than with the 10 day regimen. This result was unexpected since the 10 day regimen was designed as a more aggressive continuous attack on malignant cells in the CSF, covering many potential tumor doublings. Possible explanations for this result put forward by the investigators were tumor enhancing properties of long term citrovorum factor (all patients received IM leucovorin with IT methotrexate), interference with host defense mechanisms due to long term methotrexate, new tumor cells introduced by multiple LP's, or methotrexate resistance. Contradictory results may be due to the extreme sensitivity of Burkitt's to methotrexate thus not requiring many IT methotrexate administrations to eradicate. Thus, giving more IT methotrexate injections than necessary, possibly allows the emergence of others factors as described above.

Further studies involved treatment of 31 episodes of malignant pleocytosis in 38 patients utilizing 4 different Ara-C regimens as outlined in Table II. The patients that received the Ara-C 10-50 mg qw x 4 and the Ara-C 30 mg qd x 4 regimens had been previously treated with methotrexate. As can be seen, all but two patients in all of the regimens responded to IT Ara-C. The two that did not respond were in the group treated with the combination of Ara-C and methotrexate.

As in the methotrexate regimen used in Burkitt's lymphoma (reported in that section) it is suggestive that a 4 day regimen is better than the 10 day regimen in duration of CNS remission. Due to the small numbers of patients, however, it is not known whether this difference is significant.

REFERENCES

1. Janota, I. Involvement of the nervous system in malignant lymphoma in Nigeria. Brit J Cancer, 20: 47, 1966.

2. Burkitt, D.P., and Wright, D.H. Burkitt's lymphoma. Edinburg & London, E & S Livingstone, 1970.

3. Clifford, P., Surjeet, S., Stjernsward, J., and Klein, G. Long-term survival of patients with Burkitt's lymphoma: An assessment of treatment and other factors which may relate to survival. Cancer Res 27: 2578, 1967.

4. Ziegler, J.L., and Bluming, A.Z. Intrathecal chemotherapy in Burkitt's lymphoma. In Press.

VIII. AN OVERVIEW OF THERAPY OF ACUTE LEUKEMIA

From almost the inception of the modern era of chemotherapy, which began at the end of World War II, acute
lymphocytic leukemia was shown to be highly responsive
to drug therapy. The initial success against acute leukemia was achieved by Farber in 1948, when he demonstrated
that the folic acid antagonist, aminopterin, produced
complete remissions in some patients with acute leukemia[1].
Since then a variety of agents with differing mechanisms
of action have been developed which have the ability to
induce complete remission, and the combined use of these
agents, coupled with effective supportive therapy, can
result in disappearance of all evidence of disease for
more than 90% of children with acute lymphocytic leukemia.

In leukemia, the bone marrow is replaced by leukemic
cells, resulting in a marked decrease in circulating blood
of the formed elements normally produced in the marrow.
When complete remission is achieved with chemotherapy, these
blood elements increase to normal values, and the proportion
of leukemic cells in the bone marrow decreases to less than
5%. In addition, a complete remission represents a complete
abatement of the fever, infection, hemmorrhage and weakness
usually present in patients prior to treatment. The clinical
result of a complete remission is indistinguishable from
a "cure".

In Table I are listed the drugs shown capable of inducing complete remission in acute lymphocytic leukemia,
with pooled available data on file with the Cancer Therapy
Evaluation Branch. As can be seen, these represent a wide
range of drugs with differing mechanisms of action.

If chemotherapy is discontinued when the patient achieves
a complete remission, the disease will reappear rapidly, the
average duration of such unmaintained remissions being only
2 to 3 months. This would indicate that there are persistent
leukemic cells at a concentration which is lower than can
be detected by available means. The early workers found that
continuous treatment with folic acid antagonists appeared
to be a more satisfactory therapeutic technique than
deliberately allowing for a relapse between successive
remissions and then giving a repeat course. In 1963, Freireich
was the first to delineate a maintenance activity for drugs
independent of induction[2]. Previously untreated children
induced into remission with prednisone were randomly allocated to 6-mercaptopurine or placebo for maintenance. The 6-mer-
captopurine treated patients showed a three-fold increase in
remission duration over the placebo treated group, which
was statistically significant to a high degree.

Table I

AGENTS CAPABLE OF PRODUCING REMISSION IN
ACUTE LYMPHOCYTIC LEUKEMIA – POOLED DATA ON FILE WITH CTEB

Agent	Type of Agent	# Pts. eval.	# achieving CR	% CR	Median Duration (months)
Methotrexate	Antimetabolite of the vitamin folic acid	73	18	24	6
Prednisone	Adrenal cortical hormone	863	391	45	2
6-mercaptopurine	Antimetabolite of Hypoxanthine	544	189	35	6
Vincristine	Plant alkaloid	349	142	41	1.5
Cyclophosphamide	Alkylating agent	347	46	13	$\approx$3
Daunorubicin	Antibiotic	82	12	15	
L-asparaginase	Enzyme	205	101	50	1-2
Arabinosyl Cytosine	Antimetabolite inhibitor of DNA polymerase	122	9	7	

In a subsequent study, children who had relapsed from prior other treatment were induced with the combination of 6-mercaptopurine and prednisone, and then randomly allocated between 6-mercaptopurine maintenance and 6-mercaptopurine maintenance plus periodic vincristine and prednisone inducer doses[3]. The group receiving vincristine and prednisone inducer doses had considerably longer remissions. This study revealed the intial proof that the use of so-called "periodic reinduction" therapy exercises an effect on the leukemic population even though it was below the threshold of clinical detection. This observation constitutes one of the major conceptual advances made in leukemia therapy in the last decade.

Another major development has been the discovery that the use of active agents in combination is markedly superior to their use singly. When one considers the number of active agents in Table I, it is quickly apparent that only a few of the possible combinations have been tried; but in almost every case where combinations have been used they have proven

Table II
COMPARISON OF SINGLE AGENT AND COMBINATION
CHEMOTHERAPY OF ACUTE LYMPHOCYTIC LEUKEMIA
OF CHILDHOOD FOR REMISSION INDUCTION

Drugs	% CR	Reference
Vincristine	41	4
Prednisone	45	4
6-mercaptopurine	35	4
Methotrexate	24	4
Cyclophosphamide	13	4
Daunorubicin	15	4
L-asparaginase	50	4
Arabinosyl Cytosine	7	4
6-MP + prednisone	82, 86	5, 6
MTX + prednisone	80	6
Cyclophosphamide + prednisone	76	7
Vincristine + prednisone	85, 88	8, 9
Daunorubicin + prednisone	80	10
Daunorubicin + VCR + prednisone	97	11
6-MP, MTX, VCR + prednisone	88, 94	12, 13

better than the single therapy modality. Table II compares
the results with various combinations with the single agent
results in the remission induction of acute lymphocytic
leukemia. As can be seen, a variety of combinations have
been able to induce from 76-97% of patients into complete
remission, which is clearly superior to the best of single
agents.

Another major advance in leukemia therapy was the discovery of the critical importance of dosage schedule for
any given drug. Goldin, in a series of classic experiments,
demonstrated in the leukemia L1210 system that methotrexate
given every fourth day was superior to daily usage of the
drug[14]. This superiority was demonstrable only in the early
stage of the disease (soon after tumor inoculum) which might
be considered analogous to leukemia in remission. In the
late or advanced L1210, which is analogous to leukemia in
relapse, this schedule dependency difference was not seen.
This schedule sensitivity for methotrexate was then confirmed in man in a series of elegant clinical experiments
performed by the Acute Leukemia Cooperative Group B.
Methotrexate for induction therapy was randomly allocated
to a daily or intermittent twice weekly schedule, followed
by maintenance on daily or intermittent methotrexate after
re-randomization[15]. No difference was found in remission
induction (31% and 28%), although the twice weekly methotrexate schedule afforded longer remissions. This con-
firmation of the findings of Goldin was further confirmed
in a series of studies by Acute Leukemia Group B, in which

Table III
THE EFFECT OF THE SCHEDULE OF MTX
WHEN USED AS REMISSION MAINTENANCE IN CHILDHOOD ACUTE LEUKEMIA
AFTER INITIAL INDUCTION WITH VINCRISTINE + PREDNISONE
AS SHOWN BY ACUTE LEUKEMIA GROUP B (8,13,17)

Dosage and Schedule	Number of Children Treated	Median Duration of Complete Remission
3 mg/m^2/d P.O.	28	3.3
30 mg/m^2 twice weekly I.M.	25	17.0
30 mg/m^2 twice weekly I.M.	22	8.9
30 mg/m^2 twice weekly P.O.	22	10.4
12-18 mg/m^2/d x 5 I.V. repeated as soon as tolerated (3 courses)	35	5.0
3 courses as above, then 30 mg/m^2 twice weekly P.O.	57	18.5
12-18 mg/m^2/d x 5 as above for 8 months	54	10.8
12-18 mg/m^2/d x 5 for 8 months then 30 mg/m^2 twice weekly P.O.	8	>24

previously untreated children were induced with the combition of vincristine plus prednisone and then randomly allocated to various schedules of methotrexate for maintenance[8]. In the first study (#6307), the comparison was between 3 mg/m^2 daily orally and 30 mg/m^2 twice weekly intramuscularly. A highly significant difference in remission duration favoring the twice weekly parenteral methotrexate over the oral daily dose developed. This study was followed by a study (#6311), in which the importance of the route of drug administration was evaluated[16]. In this study, the randomization, after vincristine and prednisone induction, was to methotrexate 30 mg/m^2 either PO or IV. No evidence of effect of route of administration was found, leaving the proposition that the schedule was the crucial factor. The entire series of Acute Leukemia Group B's experiments with methotrexate maintenance therapy is outlined in Table III.

One of the building blocks in the strategy of designing protocols with curative intent for acute lymphocytic leukemia has been the information obtained about the residual leukemic population by observing the time of relapse after cessation of treatment. This has been used as a gross bioassay system of the (leukemocidal) effect of a given treatment. In order to accomplish this assay certain assumptions have been made, most of which are supported by a good deal of experimental data. These assumptions as elucidated by Zubrod are outlined in Table IV[18]. One of the most crucial assumptions made is the simple concept that one viable leukemic cell in a favorable anatomic site is eventually lethal and that treatment that fails to eradicate, with or without help from host defense mechanisms, every leukemic cell will fail to cure. If host defense mechanisms will eradicate some number of leukemic cells, then therapy must at least reduce the total cell population to that number.

Table IV
TREATMENT OF ACUTE LEUKEMIAS:
PRESENT ASSUMPTIONS

1. Total kill of leukemic cells required for cure.

2. Leukemic cell population of $\approx 1 \times 10^{12}$.

3. Doubling time $\approx 4 - 6$ days.

4. Exponential growth for majority of cells.

5. Exponential cell kill - logarithmic order of cell death for a given dosage of drug.

6. Combinations give greater cell kill than single agents.

In 1937, Furth and Kahn carried out single cell inocula-
tions with a micromanipulator and showed that one viable
leukemic cell can be lethal to the mouse[19]. The group at
Southern Research Institute has repeatedly confirmed this
observation[20]. They have shown that one leukemic L1210 cell,
and its progeny dividing on the average every half day,
will produce one billion (10^9) leukemic cells and kill the
host in 15 to 18 days.

Another crucial assumption made is that a given dosage
of a given drug kills the same percentage of leukemic cells
and not the same number in leukemic cell populations of
widely varying sizes[20]. This concept of constant percent
cell kill is called the "logarithmic order of cell death"
or "exponential cell kill" and is a concept discovered
around the turn of the century by bacteriologists working
with "disinfectants."

The data indicating constant percent cell kill has
raised interesting questions regarding how we can best use
the available drugs to effect total eradication of the
leukemic cell population in man. With a single dose of an
agent, the ability to produce complete cell eradication
depends on the effectiveness of a drug within dosages of
acceptable toxicity. With multiple doses of an agent, the
situation becomes more complex and factors such as the
cell-kill capability of the agent, generation time of the
cancer cells and period of recovery of the host after a
given dosage, all must be taken into consideration[21].

It has been estimated, based on the degree of organ
infiltration and organ size that a child (weighing 30 kg or
66 pounds) with acute leukemia, before treatment or after
relapse, on the average harbors about 2.5×10^{12} leukemic
cells (2,500,000,000,000)[21]. The total of 10^{12} cells represents a kilogram of leukemic cells in the average child,
10^{13} cells would represent 10 kg, which is clearly too much,
and 10^{11} leukemic cells 100 grams, which is too few. The
generation time of the acute lymphocytic leukemic cells in
humans has been estimated by Ellison and Murphy, and their
data indicates a doubling time of about 4 to 5 days[22].

Utilizing a complicated formula and assuming a 4-day
generation time, it has therefore been possible, utilizing
the duration of unmaintained remission, to make a rough
calculation of the cell kill achieved with a given regimen.
With vincristine alone for induction, there is a 41 day
median duration of remission[23] and this extrapolates back
to 10^9 cells remaining when therapy was stopped. Prednisone
alone gives a 60 day median duration of remission and extrapolates back to 10^8 remaining leukemic cells. Those patients
who achieved complete remission on vincristine or prednisone
have a 1000 or 10,000 fold reduction in the number of leukemic cells based on these calculations. With the "VAMP"
program at the National Cancer Institute, the median time

TABLE V
First Line Protocols of Acute Leukemia Cooperative Group B
in Acute Lymphocytic Leukemia

Protocol No.	Induction	Consolidation	Maintenance
6601	Vincristine 2 mg/m^2/wk + Prednisone a. 40 mg/m^2/d b. 120 mg/m^2/d	MTX 12, 15 or 18 mg/m^2/d x 5 IV 3 courses	a. No Treatment b. MTX 30 mg/m^2/ biw PO treat 2 yrs. from M_1 c. MTX 12, 15, 18 mg/m^2/d x 5. Treat 240 days from M_1 d. C + VCR + Pred- nisone "Periodic Reinduction"
6801	a. L-asparaginase 1000 IV/ kg/d x 5 Then VCR 2 mg/m^2/wk + Pred. 120 mg/m^2/d b. L-asparaginase. Then VCR + Pred. as in a) + Dau- norubicin 50 mg/m^2/wk IV c. Vincristine + Prednisone alone d. Daunorubicin, Vincristine + Prednisone	None	a. VCR + Pred. one week each month b. Same + MTX 30 mg/m^2/biw PO c. Same with Dau- norubicin added to VCR d. 6-MP 90 mg/m^2/d MTX 15 mg/m^2/d + VCR + Pred. as in a) e. Same as d) with Daunorubicin added
7111	a. Vincristine + Prednisone (VP) b. Vincristine + Dexamethasone 6 mg/m^2/d PO (VD) c. L-asparaginase 1000 IV/kg/d x 10 Followed by VP or VD d. L-asparaginase as above concomitantly with VP or VD e. L-asparaginase as above after 3 weeks of VP or VD	MTX 15 mg/m^2/d x 5 IM 9 day rest and repeat ↓ 6-Mercaptopurine 600 mg/m^2/d x 5 a day rest and repeat. ↓ CNS Prophylactic therapy 2400 R cranial x-ray + IT MTX vs. IT MTX alone	a. MTX and 6-MP courses as in consolidation followed by BCNU 150 mg/m^2 immed. after last dose of 6-MP b. Treatment as above to 1 year- further R_x to be determined

to relapse was 156 days which, if the above assumptions are
correct, that means that treatment reduced the number of
leukemic cells by as much as 10 logs[23].

The Acute Leukemia Group B looked at unmaintained remission after 3 intensive 5-day courses of methotrexate given
after induction with vincristine plus prednisone and cal-
culated that 120 days of therapy would be needed to achieve
complete leukemocidal effect[17]. They then designed a program
(#6601), outlined in Table V, including consolidation and
intensification treatment with repeated courses of methotrexate which deliberately lasted 240 days. For comparison
purposes there were again only three courses of methotrexate,
twice weekly methotrexate for 24 months and a regimen of
intermittent inducer doses of vincristine and prednisone
given during the 240 days of treatment ("Regimen D"). The
data from this study demonstrated that the duration of unmaintained remission after 8 months of methotrexate therapy
was longer than after 3 courses, indicating a substantially
lowered residual leukemic cell burden. In Regimen D, the
interspersing of vincristine and prednisone reinduction type
therapy lengthened the duration of remission even more.
In a small group of patients, methotrexate twice weekly
was begun after 8 months of the 5-day courses of methotrexate. This group has had an extraordinary duration of
remission and survival at last report.

The next first line protocol of Acute Leukemia Group
B (#6801 - Table V) attempted to answer the following
questions: (Lucius Sinks, personal communication):

1. Whether the combination of Daunorubicin, vincristine
    and prednisone would be more efficient than vincristine
    plus prednisone for induction of therapy.

2. Whether pretreatment with L-asparaginase before induc-
    tion with either of the above would enhance the effect.

3. To assess the relative value of reinduction treatments
    during maintenance with Daunorubicin, vincristine and
    prednisone, as compared to vincristine plus prednisone
    alone.

4. To compare maintenance treatment with methotrexate twice
    weekly alone versus methotrexate twice weekly combined
    with daily 6-mercaptopurine.

This study has been completed and the preliminary
analysis shows Daunorubicin to be of no discernable value
in combination for either induction or for periodic reinduction during maintenance. The optimal regimen appears to be
pretreatment with L-asparaginase, followed by induction
with vincristine plus prednisone and maintenance with the
combination of methotrexate and 6-mercaptopurine along

with staccato reinforcements with vincristine and prednisone[24].

The most recent protocol of Acute Leukemia Group B
(#7111) is also outlined in Table V. This complicated
protocol has the following objectives: (James Holland,
personal communication):

1.   To determine whether dexamethasone is at least equal
     to prednisone in its anti-leukemic activity and whether
     dexamethasone decreases the occurrence of infection
     and particularly fatal sepsis during the induction
     phase.

2.   To determine in untreated children if the frequency
     of remissions attained with vincristine and corti-
     costeroids can be increased by addition of asparaginase,
     and whether the position of asparaginase in the treat-
     ment schedule (before, during or after the vincristine
     and steroid) influences the remission duration.

3.   To determine the remission duration achieved with
     prolonged methotrexate and 6-mercaptopurine and BCNU
     in repeated intensive courses interspersed with periodic
     inducer doses of vincristine and steroid.

4.   To determine whether the occurrence of CNS leukemia
     can best be forestalled by the use of intensive IT
     methotrexate or the combination of radiotherapy
     to the cranium and IT methotrexate.

At the National Cancer Institute beginning in 1962,
intensive combination chemotherapy for acute lymphocytic
leukemia was pioneered by Freireich, Karon and Frei[25].
They utilized a combination of the four agents most active
in inducing complete hematological remission: methotrexate,
6-mercaptopurine, vincristine and prednisone. Each drug
was given at the dose and schedule which had been demostrated at that time to be most effective for remission
induction. The four drugs were given simultaneously over
a period of ten days. The study received the abbreviated
name "VAMP" and is fully detailed in Table VI, which out-
lines the flow of the protocols at the National Cancer
Institute over the last decade. When complete remission
was achieved, additional 10-day courses of therapy were
administered, separated by 10-day or longer intervals for
recovery from any observed toxicity. After a median of 5
such consolidation treatments given early in remission,
therapy was discontinued. Seventeen consecutive newly
diagnosed children were treated with this regimen. Eleven
children completed the consolidation treatment of 5 additional courses after induction and the median duration of
unmaintained remission was 5 months, with 9 of the 11
patients relapsing within 35 weeks.

Table VI
SEQUENCE OF FIRST LINE PROTOCOLS
FOR ACUTE LYMPHOCYTIC LEUKEMIA
AT THE NATIONAL CANCER INSTITUTE

Induction	Consolidation	Maintenance
"VAMP" Vincristine 2 mg/m^2/wk x 2 MTX 20 mg/m^2 q 4 days 6-MP 60 mg/m^2/d P.O. Prednisone 40 mg/m^2/d P.O. Course is 10-14 days	5 additional "VAMP" courses	None
"BIKE" VCR 2 mg/m^2/wk Prednisone 40 mg/m^2/d	Methotrexate 15 mg/m^2/d x 5 I.V. ↓ 9-day rest 6-mercaptopurine 1000 mg/m^2/d x 5 I.V. ↓ 9-day rest Cytoxan 1000 mg/m^2 I.V. single dose Six such cycles	None

"POMP"
VCR 2 mg/m^2/d x 1
MTX 7.5 mg/m^2/d x 5 I.V.
6-MP 600 mg/m^2/d x 5 I.V.
Prednisolone 1000 mg/m^2/d
    x 5 I.V.
Courses repeated after 9-day
    intervals
	4
	additional
	"POMP"
	courses
		"POMP"
		course
		monthly
		for 12
		months

"New POMP" "POMP" as above plus L-asparaginase 6000 I.U/m^2/d x 5 I.V.	Continued "POMP" for 6 months, then BCNU 100-150 mg/m^2 single dose	A. None B. Continued "POMP"

This study was followed by a program in which remission
was induced with the combination of vincristine and prednisone, and consolidation therapy consisted of a 5-day
course of methotrexate followed after a 9 day or longer
interval by a 5 day course of 6-mercaptopurine and another
9 day or longer interval by cyclophosphamide given in a
single dose[26].

This cycle of 3 compounds was repeated a second time
and thus the protocol was named "BIKE" because of its
bicyclic nature. This study utilized the agents individually, in sequence, and allowed the use of a full therapeutic dosage of each compound, and utilized all five of
the compounds then known to be of established value in
remission induction. After six courses of consolidation,
treatment was discontinued and the patient observed[27].
Fifteen patients entered this study and 12 completed the
consolidation treatment. The pattern of recurrence and

the duration of unmaintained remission for this study was
similar to that observed for "VAMP"[28]. It was clear that
these protocols had not eradicated the disease but that
the consolidation approach (intensive treatment after the
induction of remission) had significantly reduced the
residual leukemic load.

The "BIKE" study was followed by a third study of
intensive therapy called "POMP". It incorporated the two
major components of the preceding studies. It was a combination chemotherapy program, but the treatment was given
in higher doses for shorter periods of time. The four
active remission inducing agents (prednisone, Oncovin,
methotrexate and Purinethol) were given simultaneously
over a 5-day period, followed by 9 days of rest. The
protocol called for a median of 2 remission induction
courses followed by 4 consolidation courses of treatment
given at 2 week intervals. Unlike the "VAMP" and "BIKE"
studies, where treatment was discontinued after consolidation, a 5-day course of "POMP" was given monthly for the
next 12 months in an attempt to eliminate the leukemic
cells remaining after the consolidation treatment. This
study required over 14 months from the onset of chemotherapy
to the discontinuance of treatment. Thirty-two of 35
consecutive admissions with previously untreated acute
lymphocytic leukemia achieved complete remissions.

The "POMP" regimen resulted in longer remissions (unmaintained and maintained) and longer survival than the
low dose "VAMP" and "BIKE" regimens. Analysis of the rate
of relapse in the "POMP" study suggested that the period
during which no relapses occurred approximated the period
of intensive early treatment, and that subsequently, despite
monthly "reinductions" with the same drugs, a constant
rate of recurrence was evident[30]. This recurrence rate has
changed little at the point 14 months from the start of
the remission period when all therapy was discontinued.

The next study was entitled "New POMP" and consisted
of courses of "POMP" with the addition of L-asparaginase
to be repeated as often as possible to a point six months
following the accomplishment of remission in an attempt
to reduce the leukemic cell load. At the end of this six
month period, 1-3 bischloroethyl nitrosourea (BCNU) is
given to attack the remaining cells which may be in non-
proliferating state. At this point, randomization occurs
to no maintenance of continued therapy with "POMP". Preliminary analysis of this study indicates that duration
of remission has not been significantly improved over the
original "POMP" results (Henderson, E.J., personal communication).

The Children's Cancer Study Group A has recently completed a study in which remission induction was initially
tried with prednisone alone at dosages of either 2 or 4

Table VII
Two Selected Protocols of
Children's Cancer Study Group A

Title	Induction	Consolidation	Maintenance
"Additive Maintenance"	Prednisone 2 or 4 mg/kg/d or 8 mg/kg e.o.d. or 16 mg/kg q 4 d If not successful, VCR 0.075 mg/kg/wk x 6 If not successful, 6-MP 2.5 mg/kg/d p.o.+MTX 0.1 mg/kg/d p.o.	None	a. 56 day alternating courses 6-MP 2.5 mg/kg/d p.o. and MTX 0.1 mg/kg/d p.o. b. Same + Actinomycin D 25 gamma/kg i.v. day 28 of 6-MP course and HN_2 0.2 mg/kg i.v. day 28 of MTX course
# 903	VCR 2 mg/m^2/wk i.v. + Prednisone 60 mg/m^2/d p.o.	Methotrexate 15 mg/m^2/d x 5 q 14 D 4 courses	a. No treatment b. BCG 2 x wk x 4 wks then weekly c. MTX 30 mg/m^2/biw + VCR and Pred. as in Induction A for 1 wk each mo. x 8

mg/kg/day or 8 mg/kg every other day or 16 mg/kg once in
4 days (Table VII). If one of these regimens was not suc-
cessul in inducing remission, the patient was given a
course of vincristine and if that was not successful, remission induction was obtained by a combination of 6-mercap-
topurine and methotrexate in doses of 2.5 mg/kg/day and
0.1 mg/kg/day PO respectively. The patients were then
randomly divided into two groups. The control group received
56 day alternating courses of oral 6-MP at 2.5 mg/kg/day
and oral methotrexate at 0.1 mg/kg/day. The combination
group received in addition a dose of actinomycin D 25

TABLE VIII

		Median duration of complete remission in days	
	Number	Control	Combination
Entire group	135	390	478.5=16 months
Patients induced with Prednisone only	104	406	720=24 months
Patients induced with VCR or 6-MP+MTX after failing Prednisone induction	31	271	270

gamma/kg IV on day 28 of the 6-MP course and nitrogen mustard 0.2 mg/kg IV on day 28 of the methotrexate course. The results are outlined in Table VIII.[31]

This study leads to the important conclusion that we may be neglecting the potential role of a variety of agents either discarded for acute lymphatic leukemia in the 1950's or never fully evaluated, such as actinomycin D, nitrogen mustard and the fluorinated pyrimidines.

This study was followed by another study in which after a methotrexate + prednisone induction randomization is to six maintenance arms including the two above plus one with actinomycin D during both 56 day maintenance regimens, one with nitrogen mustard during both regimens, one reversing the actinomycin D and nitrogen mustard from the first study and one utilizing 5-fluorouracil 10 mg/kg on day 28 of both the 6-MP and methotrexate course. The results of the study have not yet been reported in the literature but long term remissions are being seen (Dennis Hammond, personal communication).

The new protocol of Children's Cancer Study Group A is outlined in Table VII and involves treatment with vincristine, prednisone and methotrexate followed by nonspecific immunotherapy with the Bacillus of Calmette and Guerin (BCG). The purpose of this study is to evaluate the potential usefulness of this nonspecific immunotherapy in prolonging an unmaintained complete remission induced by chemotherapy and to compare the effect of the BCG immunotherapy early and late in complete remission (Myron Karon, personal communication).

Several investigators (but most prominently Mathé) have demonstrated that immunotherapy can prolong survival in the mouse leukemic model L1210[32]. Studies in man untilizing BCG[33] and killed leukemic cell preparations[34] have indicated an apparent prolongation of unmaintained remission in acute human leukemia. Experiments in animals have indicated that immunotherapy of the BCG type is not effective unless the original leukemic cell population can be significantly reduced to approximately 10^5 cells. It has not been proven that this is true in man, but it would appear likely.

The studies from St. Jude's Hospital, which will be described in a later chapter, have also achieved striking results, including a high percentage of children remaining free of disease for five years or longer.

In summary, the available chemotherapy for acute lymphocytic leukemia in children has demostrated great selectivity and specificity for the tumor over the host. More than 90% of patients can be returned to a condition of completely normal health indicated by a complete hematological remission. With the advanced concepts of

intensification or consolidation, prophylactic therapy
of the central nervous system and prolonged maintenance
with periodic reusage of induction type therapy, 5 year
survivors are no longer a rarity and to speak about cure
is no longer utopian.

REFERENCES

1. Farber, S., Diamond, L.K., and Mercer, R.D. New Eng J
    Med 238: 787, 1948.

2. Freireich, E.J., Gehan, E., Frei, E., III, Schroeder,
    L.R., Wolman, I.J., Anbari, R., Bugert, E.O., Mills,
    S.D., Pinkel, D., Selawry, O.S., Moon, J.H., Gendel,
    B.R., Spurr, C.L., Storrs, R., Haurani, F., Hoogstraten,
    B., Lee, S. The effect of 6-mercaptopurine on the
    duration of steroid-induced remissions in acute leu-
    kemia: a model for evaluation of other potentially
    useful therapy. Blood 21: 699, 1963.

3. Chevalier, L., Glidewell, O. Schedule of 6-MP and
    effect of inducer drugs on remission maintenance in
    acute leukemia. Proc Amer Assn Cancer Res 8: 10, 1967.

4. Livingstone, R.B. and Carter, S.K. Single Agents in
    Cancer Chemotherapy. New York-Washington-London,
    IFI/Plenum, 1970.

5. Frei, E., III and Freireich, E.J. Progress and per-
    spectives in the chemotherapy of acute leukemia. In
    "Advances in Chemotherapy." New York, Acad Press,
    Inc. 2: 269, 1968.

6. Krivit, W., Brubaker, C., Thatcher, L.G., Pierce, M.,
    Perrin, E., and Hartmann, J.R. Maintenance therapy
    in acute leukemia of childhood. Comparison of cyclic
    vs. sequential methods. Cancer 21: 352, 1968.

7. Fernback, D.J., Griffith, K.M., Haggard, M.E., Holcomb,
    T.M., Sutow, W.W., Nietti, T.J. and Windmiller, J.
    Chemotherapy of acute leukemia in childhood. Comparison
    of cyclophosphamide and mercaptopurine. New Eng J Med
    275: 451, 1966.

8. Acute Leukemia Group B. New treatment schedule with
    improved survival in childhood leukemia. JAMA 194:
    75, 1965.

9. George, P., Hernandez, K., Hustu, O., Borella, L.,
    Holton, C. and Pinkel, D. A study of "total therapy"
    of acute lymphocytic leukemia in children. J Pediat
    72: 399, 1968.

10. Howard, J.P., and Tan, C. Combined daunomycin-pred-
    nisone inductions in acute leukemia. Proc Amer Assn
    Cancer Res 8: 32, 1967.

11. Bernard, J., Boiron, M., Jacquillat, C., and Weil, M. Rubidomycin in 400 patients with leukemias and other malignancies. (Abstract). Twelfth Congr Int Soc Hemat p.5, 1968.

12. Freireich, E.J., Henderson, E.S., and Frei, E., III. The treatment of acute leukemia considered with respect to cell population kinetics. In "Proliferation and spread of neoplastic cells. M.D. Anderson Hospital Symposium." Baltimore, Williams & Wilkins, 1968.

13. Henderson, E.S. Combination chemotherapy of acute lymphocytic leukemia of childhood. Cancer Res 27: 2570, 1967.

14. Goldin, A., Venditti, J.M., Humphreys, S.R. and Mantel, N. Modification of treatment schedules in the management of advanced mouse leukemia with amethopterin. J Nat Cancer Inst 17: 203, 1956.

15. Selawry, O.S. and James, D. Therapeutic index of methotrexate as related to dose schedule and route of administration in children with acute lymphocytic leukemia. Proc Amer Assn Cancer Res 6: 54, 1965.

16. Acute Leukemia Group B. Acute lymphocytic leukemia in children. Maintenance therapy with methotraxate administered intermittently. J Amer Med Assn 207: 923, 1969.

17. Holland, J.F., and Glidewell, O. Complimentary chemotherapy in acute leukemia. Recent Results in "Cancer Research." New York, Springer-Verlag, 30: 95, 1970.

18. Zubrod, C.G. Treatment of acute leukemias. Cancer Res 27: 2557, 1967.

19. Furth, J., and Kahn, M.C. The transmission of leukemia of mice with a single cell. Amer J Cancer 31: 276, 1937.

20. Skipper, H.E., Schabel, F.M., Jr. and Wilcox, W.S. Experimental evaluation of potential anti-cancer agents. XIII. On the criteria and kinetics associated with "curability" of experimental leukemia. Cancer Chemother Rep 35: 1, 1964.

21. Zubrod, C.G., Schepartz, S., Leiter, J., et al. The Chemotherapy program of the National Cancer Institute: history, plans and analysis. Cancer Chemother Rep 50: 349, 1966.

22. Ellison, R.B. and Murphy, M.L. Apparent doubling time of leukemic cells in marrow. (Abstract). Clin Res 12: 284, 1964.

23. Frei, E., III, and Freireich, E.J. Progress and perspectives in chemotherapy of acute leukemia. In "Advances in Chemotherapy" (Goldin, A., Hawking, F., and Schnitzer, R.J., eds.). New York, Academic Press, Inc. 2: 269, 1965.

24. Glidewell, O.J., and Holland, J.F. Clinical trials of the Acute Leukemia Group B in acute lymphocytic leukemia. Presented at the 5th International Symposium on comparative leukemia research, 1971. (In press).

25. Freireich, J., Karon, E.M., and Frei, E., III. Quadruple combination therapy (VAMP) for acute lymphocytic leukemia in childhood. (Abstract). Proc Amer Assn Cancer Res 5: 20, 1964

26. Freireich, E.J., Karon, M., Flatow, F., and Frei, E., III. Effect of intensive cyclic chemotherapy (BIKE) on remission duration in acute lymphocytic leukemia. (Abstract). Proc Amer Assn Cancer Res 6: 20, 1965.

27. Frei, E., III, and Freireich, E.J. Progress and perspectives in the chemotherapy of acute leukemia. In "Advance in Chemotherapy." (Goldin, A., Hawking, F. and Schnitzer, R.J., eds.). New York, Academic Press, Inc. 2: 269, 1965.

28. Freireich, E.J., Henderson, E.S., and Frei, E., III. The proliferation and spread of neoplastic cells. M.D. Anderson Symposium. Baltimore, the Williams and Wilkins Co., 1968.

29. Henderson, E.S., Freireich, E.J., Karon, M., and Rosse, W. High dose combination chemotherapy in acute lymphocytic leukemia of childhood. (Abstract). Cancer Res 7: 30, 1966.

30. Henderson, E.S. Combination chemotherapy of acute lymphocytic leukemia of childhood. Cancer Res 27: 2570, 1967.

31. Leiken, S., Brubaker, C., Hartmann, J., et al. The use of combination therapy in leukemia remission. Cancer 24: 427, 1969.

32. Mathé, G. Rev Franc Etud Clin Biol 12: 912, 1967.

33. Mathé, G., et al. Lancet 1: 697, April 5, 1969.

34. Skrkovich, S.V., Kisljack, N.S., Machonova, L.A., and Begunenko, S.A. Nature 223: 509, 1969.

IX. PROPHYLAXIS AND "TOTAL THERAPY"
OF MENINGEAL LEUKEMIA

Up to now we have seen the results of specific modes
of therapy which have been used in the treatment of meningeal leukemia. It soon becomes apparent, when reviewing
the data of each mode of therapy, that the ideal type of
therapy remains to be found. We have found that the results
of systemic chemotherapy alone in the treatment of meningeal
leukemia meets with little success giving an overall response rate in the small number of patients so treated of
$\simeq$ 27%. Lumbar puncture alone, although effective in relieving the symptoms of intracranial pressure in $\simeq$ 40-
50% of the cases cannot be considered as the ultimate form
of chemotherapy, for indeed it is only palliative. Intrathecal applications of drugs results in responses in
$\simeq$ 60-90% of patients, with Ara-C giving about a 56% response rate, methotrexate $\simeq$ 82%, and aminopterin $\simeq$ 98%.
The combination of IT Ara-C and methotrexate yields a
response rate of $\simeq$ 90%. Craniospinal irradiation seems to
be the best of the radiotherapy regimens, yielding a
response rate of $\simeq$ 92% in Sullivan's et al series when
1000 rads were used[1]. For IT therapy + radiotherapy the
percent response is $\simeq$ 85% and the median duration of
remission is about three months.

The immediate question which one must ask is what is
ideal therapy for the patient with meningeal leukemia?
To answer this question it seems worthwhile to discuss the
role of prophylaxis of meningeal leukemia with either IT
methotrexate or craniospinal irradiation, modalities which
have both shown to be effective in the treatment of the
disease. We have reviewed the data separately and will
discuss IT chemotherapy/prophylaxis, radiotherapy/
prophylaxis, and then both therapies as prophylaxis for
meningeal leukemia.

As was outlined in previous sections, IT methotrexate
will yield $\simeq$ 90% response rate in the therapy of meningeal leukemia. Since the blood-brain barrier appears to
be a sanctuary for leukemic cells, one wonders what the
effect of prophylaxis with IT methotrexate would be on
the eventual outcome of the disease. Both BCNU and IT
methotrexate have been used in the attempted prophylaxis
of meningeal leukemia. Several studies have combined such
prophylaxis with an organized regimen for systemic therapy
in an attempt to prolong remission duration.

There have been several reports on the use of IT
methotrexate both in the induction phase of treatment as
well as in the maintenance phase of treatment for the

prophylaxis against meningeal leukemia. Melhorn[2] utilized the drug in a controlled randomized study where 47 patients, with newly diagnosed acute leukemia, either received IT methotrexate, or did not, immediately after the diagnosis of systemic disease. Four of the 47 patients were found to have CNS involvement at the time of the original spinal tap and were given IT methotrexate and removed from subsequent study groups. Of the remaining 43 patients, 24 received a single dose 0.9 mg/kg of methotrexate IT within 24 hours of the original diagnosis of systemic disease, while 19 patients acted as controls and received no chemo-prophylaxis. Follow-up studies of the CSF were done when clinical signs and symptoms suggested meningeal involvement. Thirteen patients in each group developed meningeal leukemia (54.2% of 24 patients in the treated group; 68.4% of 19 patients in the control group). The difference in the percentage involvement was not considered significant. Average time to onset of CNS involvement in the treated patients was 11.9 months, compared to 7.6 months for the untreated group. This difference was statistically significant. Unfortunately no data was given on the effect of such therapy on the duration of systemic remission or survival.

Frei et al[3] was one of the first to employ IT methotrexate during the maintenance phase in the treatment of ALL. A summary of their experimental design is shown on Table I.

There was no intensive phase and craniospinal irradiation is not used early in remission. However, prophylactic CNS therapy was given at one week into remission under Section III of the protocol and then carried out at monthly intervals. Eighty-two percent of the patients achieved a complete remission. The median duration of remission was ≃ 7 1/2 months. The duration of remission was not affected by IT methotrexate at monthly intervals. However, the incidence of meningeal leukemia was ≈ 17% in Programs I and II but only 3% in treatment Program III.

Similar findings have also been seen by other investigators. Spevak[4], in 1964, found that prophylactic IT methotrexate at monthly intervals yielded a median survival of 18.5 months and only a 10% incidence of meningeal leukemia. Unfortunately this study was not controlled so whether the IT methotrexate directly influenced the remission duration, or decreased the incidence of meningeal leukemia, cannot be determined.

Sullivan and her colleagues[5], in the Southwest Chemotherapy Group, just reported on a study in which the duration of CNS remissions (following initial intrathecal therapy with methotrexate) were compared between no prophylactic therapy, BCNU therapy every two months, and IT methotrexate every two months. She found that the

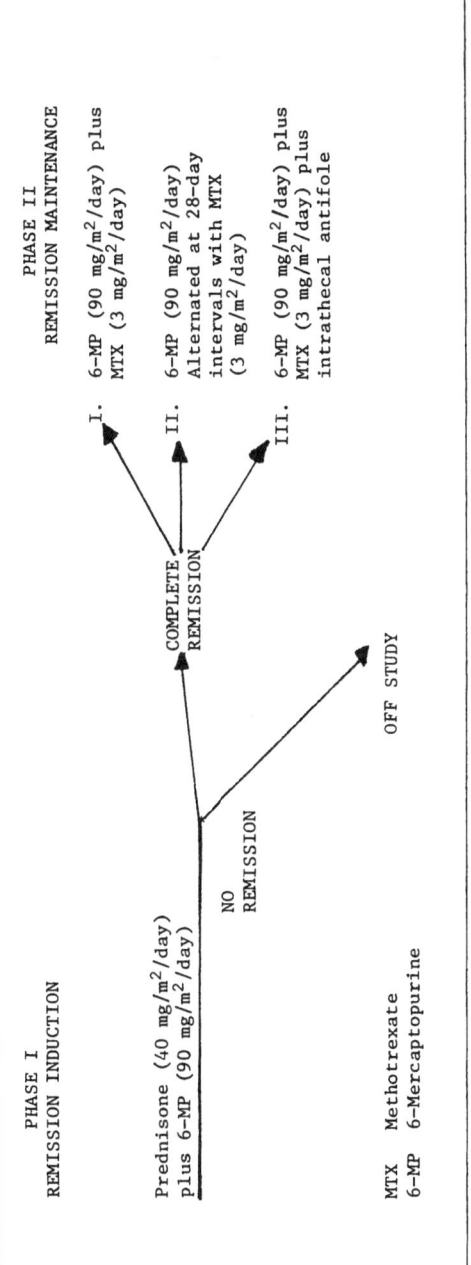

TABLE I
Experimental Design[3]

median duration of CNS remission for the no therapy group
and the BCNU therapy group was ≃ 4 months and 3 months
respectively. However, for the IT methotrexate treated
group, the median duration of CNS remission was ≃ 16 months.
However, these findings were in patients in which an
original CSF remission had been obtained with IT methotrexate. They concluded that "the superiority of the
methotrexate regimen is of such degree that it should be
considered for all patients with CNS leukemia after remission is achieved". Thus, IT methotrexate used every two
months has a definite advantage over no IT prophylactic
therapy in maintaining a CNS remission. Since this regimen
was not associated with increased morbidity or toxicity,
further investigations are currently being carried out.

It is of interest to follow the rationale and results
of the St. Judes Hospital Chemotherapy Group, and other
investigators in the field, in their use of combined chemotherapy and radiotherapy in the prophylaxis against and
treatment of CNS leukemia in man. We would also like to
propose a rational protocol for the treatment of leukemia
and CNS leukemia as derived from these and other investigators.

Over the past 8 years, Pinkel and his associates have
been using "total therapy" in the treatment of ALL in children. The first pilot study[6] (Total Therapy I) was accomplished with three children in which remission induction
with prednisone (Pred) and vincristine (VCR) was followed
by daily 6-mercaptopurine (6-MP) orally and weekly VCR and
Cytoxan (CTX) IV. During early remission, 500 rads of Co^{60}
were administered to the entire craniospinal axis. The

TABLE II
Total Therapy III for Children with Acute Lymphocytic Leukemia[8]

DESIGN OF THE STUDY

PHASE I
Remission Induction

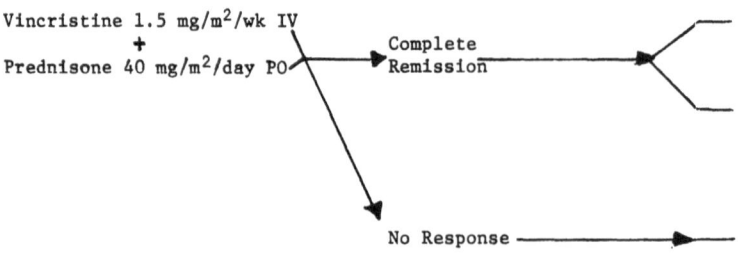

PHASE I
Remission Induction: Vincristine 1.5 mg/m²/wk IV + Prednisone 40 mg/m²/day PO → Complete Remission / No Response

next 12 children were entered in the second pilot study[7] which utilized VCR and Pred for induction (Total Therapy II). On this regimen 10/12 went into 'complete remission. They were subsequently treated with either daily 6-MP or weekly methotrexate combined with VCR and CTX administered every two weeks. This group of patients also received craniospinal irradiation with 500 rads of Co^{60}. In these two groups of patients, the median duration of complete remission was 8 months and the median survival was 20 months with two patients surviving five years or more.

On the basis of this data and the data which was being accrued by other investigators in the field, Pinkel and his associates designed a study (Total Therapy III), that could incorporate an intensive phase and a maintenance phase after remission induction as outlined in Table II[8]. There were 31 patients in this treatment group. Twenty-seven children (87%) achieved complete remission in a median time of 28 days. The median duration of remission and median survival were about double the previous pilot studies being 19.5 months and 34 months respectively. Five patients were still living by 5 years. Central nervous system relapse preceded hematological relapse in 12 patients; while in an additional patient, CNS relapse followed a hematological relapse. The overall incidence of central nervous system leukemia was 46% which was not smaller than that reported in previous studies from the group. The time from diagnosis to the onset of CNS leukemia ranged from 7 to 31 months with a median of $\simeq$ 17 months. Thus, by incorporating an intensive phase, being more vigorous with maintenance therapy, and increasing the dose of CNS radiation, the survival of this group of children was almost doubled.

TABLE II
Total Therapy III for Children with Acute Lymphocytic Leukemia[8]

DESIGN OF THE STUDY

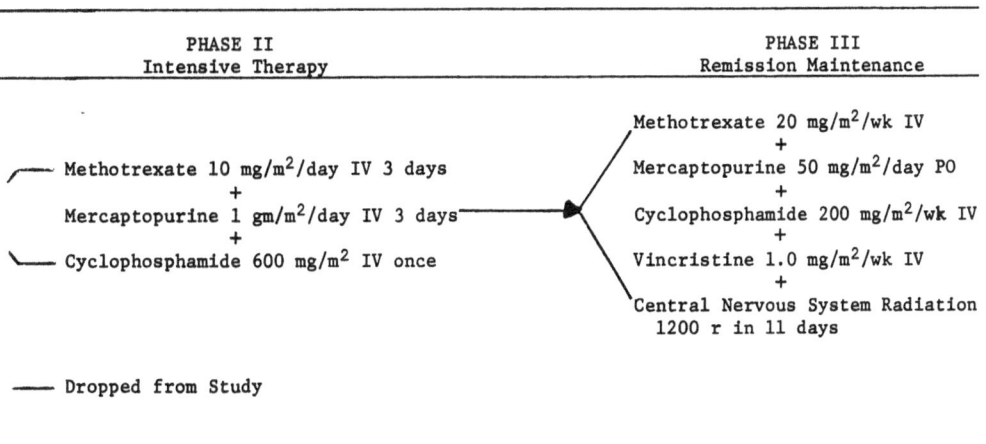

PHASE II Intensive Therapy	PHASE III Remission Maintenance
Methotrexate 10 mg/m²/day IV 3 days + Mercaptopurine 1 gm/m²/day IV 3 days + Cyclophosphamide 600 mg/m² IV once	Methotrexate 20 mg/m²/wk IV + Mercaptopurine 50 mg/m²/day PO + Cyclophosphamide 200 mg/m²/wk IV + Vincristine 1.0 mg/m²/wk IV + Central Nervous System Radiation 1200 r in 11 days

—— Dropped from Study

However, central nervous system radiation by the method and dosage used had no influence on the development of CNS leukemia.

To further study the effects of the changes in the Total Therapy III protocol, a fourth study was carried out, Total Therapy IV, where drugs were either administered in full dosages or half dosages during the maintenance phase and craniospinal irradiation was left out altogether[9]. The general schema of this protocol is illustrated in Table III. This protocol was designed to answer the question as to whether high doses of the multiple antileukemic drugs were necessary for optimal maintenance of remissions. By eliminating the CNS radiation, this protocol also helped answer another question as to whether craniospinal radiation given during early remission prolonged the interval between diagnosis and the development of CNS leukemia. In answer to the first question, the median duration of complete remission was 15 months (as it had been in Total Therapy II) for those receiving the full dosages. However, in those patients receiving 1/2 dosages during the maintenance phase, the median duration of complete remission was only 6 months. Also the survival in the patients receiving the 1/2 dose therapy was 21 months; while the survival of those receiving full doses of chemotherapeutic agent

TABLE III
Total Therapy IV [9]

TREATMENT PLAN

Phase	Purpose	Duration	Drug Schedule
1	Remission induction	4 to 6 weeks	VCR, 1.5 mg/m^2/week, IV
			Pred. 40 mg/m^2/day, PO
2	Intensive chemotherapy	1 week	MTX, 10 mg/m^2/day x 3, IV
			MP, 1 gm/m^2/day x 3, IV
			Cyclo, 600 mg/m^2/day x 1, IV
3	Continuation	3 years or to hematological relapse	MP, 50 mg/m^2/day, PO
			MTX, 20 mg/m^2/weeks, IV
			Cyclo, 200 mg/m^2/week, IV
			VCR, 1 mg/m^2/week, IV or half-dosage of above drugs

Pinkel
VCR - Vincristine
Pred - Prednisone
MTX - Methotrexate
MP - Mercaptopurine
Cyclo - Cyclophosphamide

was ≃ 34 months. Thus, the absence of CNS radiation did not appreciably alter either remission duration or survival when compared with the results of Total Therapy III.

In answer to the second question as to the prophylactic effect of CNS radiation in the early phase of remission, a clear-cut effect was noted. As will be recalled, the median time from diagnosis to the onset of meningeal leukemia in Total Therapy III was ≃ 17 months with 46% of the children developing CNS leukemia. In Total Therapy IV, under that section that utilized the same dosages as in Total Therapy III (full dosages), the median time from diagnosis to onset of meningeal leukemia and only ≃ 11 months in 15/21 (71%) patients in which CNS leukemia developed. Thus CNS leukemia was delayed and its incidence reduced by the administration of prophylactic radiotherapy in Total Therapy III. That systemic therapy also played a role in delaying the onset of meningeal leukemia was evident by comparing the median time from diagnosis to onset of meningeal leukemia of those at the half dosage and full dosage schedule. In those patients who only received 1/2 dosage during the maintenance phase, 20/21 (95%) developed CNS leukemia in a median time of 5-7 months. Thus, development of meningeal leukemia was directly responsible for the decrease in the median time of complete remissions. All the subsequent protocols have included CNS prophylaxis either with radiotherapy alone or in combination with IT methotrexate.

Total Therapy V (outlined in Table IV) utilizes the same induction therapy as in the two previous protocols[10]. The intensive phase differs only by the addition of prednisone. During early remission, and just after the intensive phase however, a 2 1/2 week phase of CNS prophylaxis is added which includes radiotherapy to the skull (2500 r), IT methotrexate 12 mg/m^2/wk x 5 doses (with leucovorin protection systemically), and prednisone 10 mg/m^2/day orally x 7 days. The maintenance is similar to the previous full dosage protocol but is interrupted at 10 week intervals by VCR and Pred reinductions. In the previous study, complete remissions have been most often terminated by nervous system leukemia occurring in the presence of hematological remission. This present therapy schema was designed to explore the possibility that CNS leukemia and thus early termination of complete remission could be prevented by administering a moderately high dose of cranial radiotherapy along with IT methotrexate early during complete remission.

The results at this time are currently superior to those of any previous treatment program. Complete remissions were successfully attained in 32 of 35 patients (91%) entering this study. Twenty-one of the 32 children who attained remission (64%) are currently in continuous complete remissions for 23 to 30 months (median 25 months).

TABLE IV
Total Therapy V[10]

Phase 1 - Induction (4-6 wks)

Pred 40 mg/m^2/d orally x 28 to 42 d

VCR 1.5 mg/m^2/wk IV x 4 to 6 wk

Phase 2 - Intensive (1wk)

6 MP 1 gm/m^2/d IV x 3

MTX 10 mg/m^2/d IV x 3

Cyclo 600 mg/m^2/d IV x 1

Pred 20 mg/m^2/d orally x 7

Phase 3 - CNS (2 1/2 wks)

Radiotherapy Skull 2500 r

MTX IT 12 mg/m^2/2x/wk x 5 doses

Leucovorin IM, 12 mg/m^2/2x/wk x 5 doses

Pred 10 mg/m^2/d orally x 7

Phase 4 - Continuation (2 yrs)

6 MP 50 mg/m^2/d orally

MTX 20 mg/m^2/wk IV

Cyclo 200 mg/m^2/wk IV

At week No. 10 and every 10 weeks thereafter

Pred 40 mg/m^2/d orally x 15 d

VCR 1.5 mg/m^2/wk IV x 3 doses

Of ten children who received all phases of therapy (two did not due to sepsis in one and varicella in another) and who relapsed from complete remission, only three of these developed nervous system leukemia before hematological relapse and three after hematological relapse. Thus only 6 out of 32 (19%) children developed CNS leukemia as compared to ≈ 71% in the previous study. The time from diagnosis to onset of meningeal leukemia cannot be determined from the data given. The greater intensity of the CNS therapy in this study may be responsible not only for the reduction of incidence of CNS leukemia, but also for the substantial increase in the duration of complete remission.

Total Therapy VI, from the St. Jude's group, is outlined in Table V[11,12]. Total Therapy VI is designed to determine the influence of a one week course of high dose intensive chemotherapy on the duration and quality of

Table V
Total Therapy VI

Remission Induction (4-6 weeks)[11,12]
Pred 40 mg/m^2/d orally x 28 to 42 d
VCR 1.5 mg/m^2/wk IV x 4 to 6 wks
Dauno 25 mg/m^2/wk IV x 4 to 6 wks

CR MARROW
Randomize into 2 groups
1/2 Patients - GROUP A   1/2 Patients - GROUP B

Intensive Chemotherapy (7 days)   No Intensive Chemotherapy

6-MP 1 gm/m^2/d IV x 3 d
  followed by
MTX 10 mg/m^2/d IV x 3 d   NO
  followed by   DELAY
Cyclo 600 mg/m^2/d IV x 1 d

2 week delay

CONTINUATION THERAPY (3 years)

6-MP 50 mg/m^2/d orally
MTX 20 mg/m^2/ weekly orally*
Cyclo 200 mg/m^2 weekly orally*
At day 70 of this phase add:
VCR 1.5 mg/m^2/wk IV x 3 doses (days 1,8,15)
Pred 40 mg/m^2/ orally x 15 days

VCR-pred course repeated 70 days after final dose of VCR-pred of
each previous course.

Four weeks after achieving M-1 marrow patients randomized into
Group A (2 subgroups) and Group B (2 subgroups.).

GROUP A		GROUP B	
A-1 (1/4 patients)	A-2 (1/4 patients)	B-1 (1/4 patients)	B-2 (1/4 patients)
Craniospinal Radiotherapy, 2400 r	Craniospinal Radiotherapy, 2400 r when CNS leukemia develops.	Craniospinal Radiotherapy, 2400 r immediately.	Craniospinal Radiotherapy, 2400 r when CNS leukemia develops.

---

subsequent chemotherapy-maintained remissions, and evaluate the role of prophylactic craniospinal irradiation in preventing meningeal leukemia and thereby maintaining complete remissions for a longer period of time. The results of this protocol were recently reported[11,12]. A total of 94 patients were randomly allocated between craniospinal irradiation 2400 r Co^{60} and no prophylactic therapy and intensive chemotherapy or no intensive chemotherapy. All subsequently received identical multiple drug chemotherapy for at least one year. To date there is no difference between the intensive and no intensive chemotherapy. However, the prophylactic CNS radiotherapy section of the protocol already shows a marked difference. CNS leukemia has ended remission in 27 of 49 children (51%) not receiving irradiation prophylactically compared to

only 2 of 45 (6.6%) who received craniospinal irradiation
prophylactically. In 7 patients in the irradiated group,
the bone marrow was the initial site of relapse, while
one patient in this group subsequently had a bone marrow
relapse following CNS leukemia. In the non-irradiated
group, 5 systemic relapses occurred before CNS relapse,
while 3 occurred after it. Thus, both groups had the
same number (8) of bone marrow relapses. Only 4 of 45
patients in the irradiated group had reduction of radiation dosage due to toxicity. Preferentially, chemotherapy was reduced to permit completion of radiotherapy within 4 weeks. The authors concluded that "in
children with ALL receiving combination chemotherapy,
craniospinal irradiation early in remission delays or
prevents CNS leukemia."

Outlined in Table VI is the most recent St. Jude's
protocol, Total Therapy VII[13]. Total Therapy VII will
compare the efficacy and toxicity of two therapeutic
regimens given early in remission for prophylaxis of
nervous system leukemia and thereby for prolongation of
continuous complete remissions: (1) cranial radiotherapy
plus IT methotrexate; (2) craniospinal radiotherapy. It
will also determine the efficacy and toxicity of a 15
day course of prednisone and vincristine every 12 weeks
during continuation therapy in prolonging continuous
complete remissions.

Total Therapy VII will help to answer the role that
prophylactic IT methotrexate will play in reducing the
number of CNS relapses but remains deficient in one important aspect. That aspect is the role that prophylactic
IT methotrexate given continuously during the maintenance
phase would play. Indeed the St. Jude's group has yet to
explore this possibility.

We would like to propose a general protocol (Table VII)
in general terms that could integrate CNS prophylaxis into
the current concepts of remission induction and maintenance
being used today. It is a synthesis of the schema used by
Pinkel and associates and of the knowledge gained through
reviewing this subject.

First, due to the importance of maintaining systemic
remission for increased survival, we have incorporated
an intensive course of chemotherapy which is currently
divided into three phases remission induction, consolidation, and maintenance. Such a treatment schedule has been
giving the best results not only in the hands of the St.
Jude's group, but also in the other cooperative group
studies. Vincristine and prednisone is used solely for
induction since it is during this phase that the patients
will be receiving intensive CNS prophylaxis. Consolidation
as well as maintenance could be with whatever drugs cur-

TABLE VI
OUTLINE OF TOTAL THERAPY STUDY VII [13]

PHASE 1: REMISSION INDUCTION (4-6 wks)
Pred 40 mg/m^2/d orally (P.O.)
VCR 1.5 mg/m^2/ wk intravenously (I.V.)

If still either M-2 or M-3 by day 42, DROP FROM STUDY.

If patient shows progressive leukemia at any time of PHASE 1, chemotherapy will be changed in his best interest.

If in REMISSION (M-1 marrow), randomization by CARD-ENVELOPE THECHNIQUE into 4 GROUPS (CM, CMVP, CS and CSVP) for further therapy with no delay (Phase II-A and B).

CM = CRANIAL RADIATION + METHOTREXATE (MTX) INTRATHECALLY (IT)

CMVP = CM + Pred-VCR PULSE

CS = CRANIO-SPINAL RADIATION

CSVP = CS + Pred-VCR PULSE

PHASE II-A: PROPHYLAXIS OF CENTRAL NERVOUS SYSTEM (CNS) LEUKEMIA
(2 1/2 or 4 wks)

CM and CMVP - 2 1/2 wks: CRANIAL RADIATION - 2400 r
MTX - 12 mg/m^2/twice wk X 5 IT

CS and CSVP - 4 wks: CRANIO-SPINAL RADIATION - 2400 r

PHASE II-B: CONTINUATION CHEMOTHERAPY
(2-3 yrs)

All groups (CM, CMVP, CS and CSVP):

6-MERCAPTOPURINE (6-MP) - 50 mg/m^2/d P.O.

CYCLOPHOSPHAMIDE (Cyclo) - 200 mg/m^2/wk P.O.

METHOTREXATE (MTX) - 20 mg/m^2/wk P.O.

Groups CM and CMVP receive no P.O. MTX during cranial radiation with IT MTX.

PHASE III: VCR-PRED PULSE

Groups CMVP and CSVP starting on day 70 after M-1 marrow and every 12 wks from the start of the preceding pulse:

PRED - 40 mg/m^2/d x 15 days P.O.

VCR - 1.5 mg/m^2/wk x 3 doses I.V.

---

rently appear to be the most efficacious. (Currently combinations of cell cycle sensitive agents such as methotrexate and 6-MP plus a cell cycle insensitive agent such as Cytoxan). Although the inclusions of a consolidation phase showed no effect on the course of subsequent CNS disease in St. Jude's Total Therapy VI, we feel that the data are too preliminary to tell anything about systemic remission duration. From several studies to date, there is no doubt that remission maintenance with chemotherapeutic agents prolongs survival.

TABLE VII
Protocol for the Treatment of ALL in Children with
Emphasis on CNS Prophylaxis

Phase 1 - Induction (4-6 wks)
Pred 40 mg/m^2/day orally x 28 to 42 days
VCR 1.5 mg/m^2/wk IV x 4-6 weeks
Craniospinal irradiation 1500 r IT MTX 12
mg/m^2/3x/week 9 doses

After M-1 Marrow   Phase 2 Intensive (1 week; consolidation)

Combination of a number of antileukemic agents used
for combination

Phase 3 Maintenance (2 years)
Combination of a number of antileukemia agents used
in maintenance. IT MTX 12 mg/m^2 IT every 2 months

Reinduction

At week ten and every ten weeks thereafter Pred
40 mg/m^2/day orally x 15 days; VCR 1.5 mg/m^2/wk
IV x 3 doses

In terms of CNS prophylaxis, several principles seem
to be emerging. First, ≃ 10% of patients will have CNS
involvement at the time of the original diagnosis[2] and
that about another third will develop meningeal leukemia
in the first three months of their disease. Thus the need
for early treatment is apparent. In view of this, we have
proposed giving the CNS prophylaxis as soon as possible
in order that the total leukemic cell population in the
CNS would be lower and give better chance of a successful
result. We have chosen a combination approach based on
Sullivan's et al[1] data and the excellent results of the
St. Jude's group. Also, based on the data of Selawry, it
would seem rational to utilize at least 8 injections for
theoretical total cell kill. Certainly controlled studies
of the efficacy of various schedules should be done to
confirm these theories. Finally, that CNS maintenance
therapy is important in maintaining CNS remissions has
been shown by Sullivan when patients were randomized between IT methotrexate maintenance and no CNS maintenance.
It was found that prophylactic IT methotrexate every two
months maintained CNS remissions almost 5 times longer
than control patients who received no prophylactic therapy.
In this way, one will be able to follow the spinal fluid
at least every two months and therapy could be changed as
needed. Retreatment for CNS relapse while on maintenance
IT methotrexate could be accomplished by further courses
of craniospinal irradiation as well as drug manipulation.
Other agents that seem most efficacious against CNS disease
are BCNU and IT cytosine arabinoside. Certainly, pyrimethamine which was used successfully in one patient with
meningeal leukemia, may be another agent which could be

used systemically for prophylaxis in place of IT methotrexate. However, we would reserve such use until after
the appropriate clinical trials have demonstrated
significant activity of the drug against meningeal leukemia
in a suficient number of patients.

REFERENCES

1. Sullivan, M.P., Vietti, T.J., Fernbach, D.J., Griffith,
    K.M., Haddy, T.B., and Watkins, W.L. Clinical inves-
    tigations in the treatment of meningeal leukemia:
    radiation therapy regimens vs conventional intrathecal
    methotrexate. Blood 34: 301, 1969.

2. Melhorn, D.K., Gross, S., Fisher, B.J., and Newman,
    A.J. Studies on the use of "prophylactic" intrathecal
    amethopterin in childhood leukemia. Blood 36: 55,
    1970.

3. Frei, E., III, et al. The effectiveness of combinations
    of antileukemic agents in inducing and maintaining
    remission in children with acute leukemia. Blood 26(5):
    642, 1965.

4. Spevak, J. The prophylaxis of meningeal leukemia with
    intrathecal methotrexate. J Iowa Med Soc 54(5): 238,
    1964.

5. Sullivan, M.P., Haggard, M.E., Donaldson, M.H., and
    Krall, J. Comparison of the prolongation of remission
    in meningeal leukemia with maintenance intrathecal
    methotrexate (IT MTX) and intravenous bis-nitrosourea
    (BCNU). Proc Amer Assoc Cancer Res 11: 77, 1970.

6. George, P., and Pinkel, D. CNS radiation in children
    with acute lymphocytic leukemia in remission. Proc
    Amer Assn Cancer Res 6: 22, 1965.

7. George, P., Hernandez, K., Borella, L., and Pinkel, D.
    "Total Therapy" of acute lymphocytic leukemia in chil-
    dren. Proc Amer Assn Cancer Res 7: 23, 1966.

8. George, P., Hernandez, K., Hustu, O., Borella, L.,
    Holton, C., Pinkel, D. A study of "total therapy" of
    acute lymphocytic leukemia in children. Ped Pharmacol
    Ther 72: 399, 1068.

9. Pinkel, D., Hernandez, K., Borella, L. et al. Drug
    dosage and remission duration in childhood lymphocytic
    leukemia. Cancer 27: 247, 1971

10. Aur, R.J.A., et al. Central nervous system therapy in
    combination chemotherapy of childhood lymphocytic
    leukemia. Blood 37(3): 272, 1971.

11. Aur, R., Hustu, H.O., Ver Zosa, M., and Simone, J. A comparative study of "prophylactic" craniospinal irradiation in 94 children with acute lymphocytic leukemia (ALL). Proc Amer Assn Cancer Res 12: 19, 1971.

12. Aur, R.J.A., Simone, J.V., Hustu, H.O., and Ver Zosa, M.S. A comparative study of central nervous system irradiation and intensive chemotherapy early in remission of childhood acute lymphocytic leukemia. Cancer in Press.

13. Aur, R.J.A. Personal Communication.

X. SUMMARY

   Thus we have followed the treatment of meningeal leukemia from the onset of chemotherapy to the present time.
Since during this time period the incidence of meningeal
leukemia has risen about ten-fold it is becoming one of
the most frequent complications of leukemia especially
in ALL in children, accounting for the termination of
complete remission in a large number of cases. For these
reasons, a specific and concerted attempt must be aimed
at its eradication. By doing this, we may hope to one day
eradicate every leukemic cell from the body of leukemic
patients.

   We have followed the results of therapy from its begin-
nings where only systemic therapy was being used, yielding
a response rate of only 27% in the limited number of patients
in which it was employed. Simple lumbar puncture alone is
only palliative, relieving the symptoms of increased intracranial pressure in ≃ 44% of patients. Thus it has been
stressed that when following the patient with CNS leukemia
both the objective CSF parameters and the subjective symptoms and signs should be followed very closely. Various
modes of IT chemotherapy have been tried with IT methotrexate yielding about an 80-90% response rate both
objectively and subjectively. Other IT drugs are also
effective but none have proven to be superior to methotrexate. For this reason, their use probably should be
limited to refractory cases unresponsive to IT methotrexate.
Radiotherapy is somewhat less effective than IT methotrexate,
relieving both objective and subjective parameters in
≃ 63% of the cases.

   Using the results of animal models and applying the
principles found to man, we have seen that the combination
of craniospinal irradiation and IT methotrexate is successful ≃ 100% of the time and yields a remission duration of
≃ 3 months, equal to that of IT methotrexate alone. Certain
investigators have used this combination for prophylaxis
and by doing so have achieved the longest complete CNS
and hematological remissions seen in children with ALL up
this point in time. Furthermore, benefits derived from the
use of continuous prophylactic IT methotrexate has been
described in some detail.

   It is the combination of aggressive systemic chemotherapy utilizing remission induction, intensive consolidation, and maintenance therapy along with prophylactic CNS
therapy in the form of initial CNS radiation and IT methotrexate followed by every other month application of IT

methotrexate that this author feels deserves the term
"Total Therapy." A protocol utilizing this type of therapy
has been proposed based on the sum total of all the reports
and results that have been amassed in both the preclinical
and clinical fields.

Thus perhaps through use of this type of protocol, the
goal of eradicating every leukemic cell can be furthered
and the concept of cure will enter into our thinking in
the therapy of leukemia.

Abd.	Abdominal
ACTH	Adrenocorticotrophic hormone
ALL	Acute lymphocytic leukemia
AML	Acute myelocytic leukemia
Ara-C	Cytosine arabinoside
Aud.	Auditory
Av.	Average
BCG	Bacillus of Calmette and Guerin
BCNU	1,3-Bis(2-chloroethyl)-1-nitrosourea
BIW	Twice weekly
CCNSC	Cancer Chemotherapy National Service Center
CCNU	1-(2-chloroethyl)-3-cyclohexyl-1-nitrosourea
Child.	Children
CLL	Chronic lymphocytic leukemia
CML	Chronic myelocytic leukemia
CNS	Central nervous system
CR	Complete remission or complete response
CSF	Cerebrospinal fluid
CTX, Cyclo	Cytoxan, cyclophosphamide
d.	Day
Dauno.	Daunorubicin
Dist.	Disturbance
DNA	Deoxyribonucleic acid
Eval.	Evaluable
F	Female
FU, 5-FU	5-Flurouracil
GI	Gastrointestinal
IC	Intracerebral
IM	Intramuscularly
IP	Intraperitoneal
IT	Intrathecal
IV	Intravenous
kg	Kilogram
M	Male
m^2	Square meter
Med.	Median
mg.	Milligram
MP, 6-MP	6-Mercaptopurine
ML	Meningeal leukemia
Mos.	Months
MTX	Methotrexate
N&V	Nausea and vomiting
NC	No change
PO	By mouth
PR	Partial remission or partial response
Pred	Prednisone
Pts.	Patients

Rel.	Relapse
Rem.	Remission
RNA	Ribonucleic acid
Rx.	Treatment
Sep.	Separation
TD	Total dose
THF	Tetrahydrofolic acid
VCR	Vincristine
WBC	White blood count
Wt.	Weight
X-RT	Radiotherapy
Yrs.	Years

INDEX